An evidence-backed, wh
managing depression, anxie

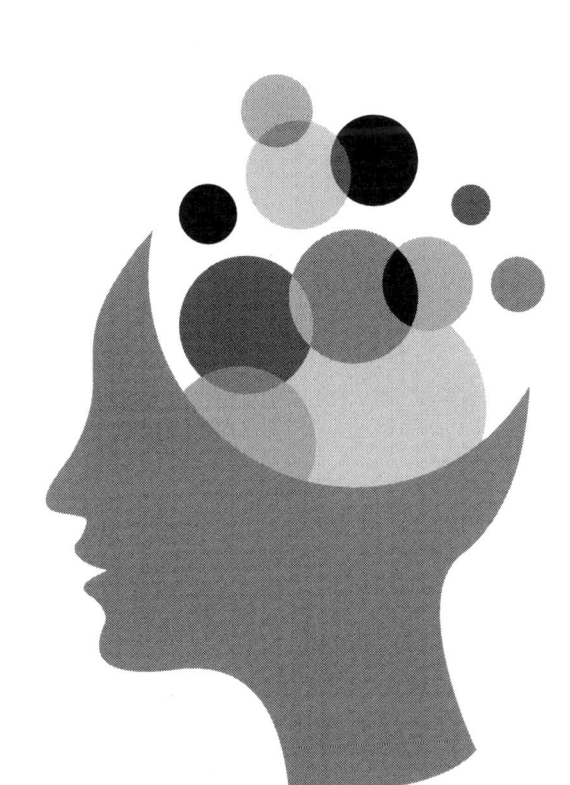

EAT YOUR BRAIN HAPPY

STEPHANIE J MOORE
MA, BSc, BA

EAT YOUR BRAIN HAPPY

*Dedicated to all of you living with or helping
those with poor mental health.
May this book bring hope and structure where
there is misery and chaos.*

First published in 2024
Copyright © Stephanie J Moore 2024. All rights reserved.
www.health-in-hand.co.uk

Paperback ISBN: 978-1-0687089-0-9

No part of this book may be reproduced, modified or transmitted in any form, or by any means, electronic or mechanical, including photocopying, reprinting, recording or any other form of information storage without the written permission of the author, except in the case of brief quotations embodied in reviews.

Every effort has been made to ensure that the information contained in the book is complete and accurate. The information and recommendations are designed to provide helpful information on the subjects discussed. This book is not meant to be used, nor should it be used, to diagnose or treat any medical condition. For diagnosis or treatment of any medical problem, consult a medical practitioner. The author is not responsible for any specific health or allergy needs that may require medical supervision and is not liable for any damages or negative consequences from any treatment, action, application or preparation, to any person reading or following the information in this book.

Should the reader choose to undertake the recommendations suggested by the author, be sure that you are taking sensible precautions and necessary medical advice. The author advises readers to take full responsibility for their safety and know their limits.

References and resources are provided for informational purposes only and do not constitute endorsement of any websites or other sources. Readers should be aware that the websites and resources listed in this book may change.

Disclaimer: The information in this book is not intended as medical advice. The author is not medically qualified and would not want anyone to stop their medications or change the dose on the basis of any of the recommendations made here. The author recommends healthy, safe adjustments to your day-to-day diet and lifestyle choices to support your body's own processes to heal and restore balance irrespective of medications. However, if you are medicated for an anxiety or depressive disorder, please speak with your prescribing doctor before taking any of the supplements mentioned here, as some may interact with medications to make them more or less potent.

STEPHANIE J MOORE

EAT YOUR BRAIN HAPPY

Contents

Thank-yous	13
About the Author	15
Preface	17
A note to the reader	19
Introduction	**21**
About this book	25
Managing expectations	26

PART ONE
YOUR BRAIN IS NOT BROKEN — 29

CHAPTER ONE
Why Is It So Hard to Be Happy? — 31

Bringing back the balance	33
What if there's no reason?	36
Anxiety: What is your body telling you?	37
Self-care for the brain	41

CHAPTER TWO
The Biology of an Unhappy Brain — 43

Happiness is a body-wide process	43
You are what you digest	45
Fuelling a happy brain	48

Fat versus sugar (ketones versus glucose) — 49
Metabolic inflexibility — 50
The insulin-resistant, 'diabetic' brain — 54
Metabolic psychiatry — 56
Taking in the sunshine — 62
Styling your life — 63

CHAPTER THREE
Inflammation — **65**
Does an inflamed body cause an unhappy brain? — 66
Managing your inflammation is managing your mental health — 69
    Anti-inflammatory practices 101 — 69

CHAPTER FOUR
Which Is in Charge, Your Gut or Your Brain? — **73**
The gut–brain dynamic — 73
Our food choices affect how we function — 77
Short-chain fatty acids: Our gut bugs' thank-you gift — 78
A short introduction to a very long nerve — 80
A poignant case history — 85

PART TWO
THE HAPPY BRAIN ACTION PLAN — **89**

CHAPTER FIVE
Your Gut Health *Is* Your Brain Health — **93**
Step 1. The big first step: Cut the junk — 93
    Refined carbs aka fast carbs and high-starch foods — 94
    Easy swaps for increasing your healthier carbs — 95
Step 2. Getting going on your gut health — 97
    Nurture your gut microbes using the 3Fs — 97
    F1: Fibre and polyphenols — 98
    How much fibre do you need? — 99
    A note on fruit — 101

Types of fibre	102
Prebiotic fibre	105
Resistant starch	107
Polyphenols	108
F2: Fermented foods	109
Types of ferments	110
Gut-friendly fermented foods	112
F3: Fasting	113
Fasting methods	116
Midnight hunger	117
Postbiotics: The power of the 3Fs combined	118

CHAPTER SIX
Happy Brain Food Day to Day — 123

The happy brain plate	125
Fibre-rich plant foods	126
Befriend bitter foods	130
Black seed oil	131
Fermented foods	133
Protein-rich foods	134
Animal-based protein	136
Look at the ingredients list	138
Plant-based protein	139
The missing link in plant proteins	140
How much protein is enough?	141
Nutrient-rich starchy foods	142
Healthy fats	144
Essential fatty acids	146
Hydration	150
Eating your brain happy	151

CHAPTER SEVEN
Unhappy Brain Foods and How to Avoid Them — 159

Highly processed foods	159

Refined grains	160
Wheat and gluten	160
Refined cooking oils	162
Alcohol	163
Sugar	164
How much sugar are you really eating?	165
Artificial sweeteners	169
Enjoy your food	172
What to do more of when eating	172
Ask yourself if you're hungry	172
Chew	173
Pause between mouthfuls	174
What to do less of when eating	174
A conscious treat	175

CHAPTER EIGHT
Strategic Supplementation — 177

Do supplements really work?	178
The basic happy brain supplement protocol	179
Multivitamin and Mineral	179
Zinc	180
Iron	180
Methylated B vitamins	181
Vitamins D_3 + K_2	185
Vitamin D_3	185
Vitamin K_2	188
Omega 3 fish oil	189
Magnesium	192
Specialist supplements	195
Vitamin C: Antioxidant, immune supporter, happy gut promoter	195
Curcumin: An anti-inflammatory superstar	197
MCT oil: Readily available brain fuel	199
Choline (citicoline): The brain booster	199
L-Taurine: The GABA-friendly amino acid	200

L-Theanine: The anxiety super-supplement ... 201
5-HTP: The depression super-supplement ... 202
Inositol: The missing B vitamin ... 202
Lithium orotate: The missing mineral ... 203
Berberine: The metabolic and gut–brain heavy hitter ... 204
Medicinal mushrooms: The future of brain health? ... 205
Herbs ... 207
Prebiotics and probiotics ... 208
    Prebiotic fibre ... 208
    Probiotics ... 210

CHAPTER NINE
Live Your Brain Happy ... **215**

Vagus nerve stimulation ... 215
    Breathing through your nose ... 217
    The basic technique ... 218
    Gargling ... 218
    Singing, vigorous humming, omming or chanting ... 219
    Full-body shaking ... 219
    Laughing and smiling ... 220
    Triggering the gag reflex ... 220
    Bilabial trill ... 221
    Cold water exposure ... 221
    Positive social connection ... 223
    Acupuncture and body work ... 223
    Red light therapy ... 224
Sleep ... 224
    Phases of sleep ... 226
    Programming sleep ... 227
    Natural light exposure in the early morning ... 227
    Daylight exposure at sunset ... 228
    Block blue light at night ... 228
    Wake and sleep times ... 229
    Magnesium ... 229

Body temperature	230
Sleep disruptors	230
Moving your body	231
Light exposure	234
Mindfulness	235
Journaling	236
Gratitude	236
Essential oils	237

Conclusion — **239**

Appendix — **243**

Recommended foods list	243
Truly super superfoods	243
Fermented foods	243
Best animal products	244
Best fats and oils	244
Best fruits	244
Best vegetables	245
Best whole grains	245
Best pulses	245
Best nuts and seeds	246
'Better than most' sweeteners	246
Resources	247
Fabulous cookbooks for a happy brain	247
Healthy eating information	247
Sites to find registered nutrition experts	248
Suppliers	248

Thank-yous

To Mr Redtenbacher for his tireless encouragement and layman's lens; to my dear friend Laura who reminded me of the importance of this book when I felt like giving up; to Goodwood Wellbeing for their unwavering belief and trust in what I do, and in particular Janet Richmond, Duchess of Richmond and Gordon, for being such a champion of my work and for providing a most glorious home at Goodwood for the gut health programme to grow and thrive; to Sally Osborn for her brilliance in making my book make sense; to Neil J Hart for his laser-like precision in making my book print-ready; to Rebecca Nicolson from New River Books for her support and guidance.

A note of deep gratitude goes to the pioneers in the compelling fields of nutritional and metabolic psychiatry who have inspired and educated me: Dr James Greenblatt, Dr Georgia Ede, Dr Chris Palmer, Dr Shebani Sethi, Dr Albert Danon, Professor Julia Rucklidge, Professor Felice Jacka and Professor Joanna Moncrieff.

Finally, thank you to all those I work with who open their hearts, bear their souls and allow me into their pain – I have learnt, and continue to learn, so much from you all.

About the Author

Stephanie has studied and worked in the integrative health field for over 30 years as a physical therapist, psychotherapist, clinical nutritionist, author and passionate educator. She combines all skill sets to help people with many kinds of health challenges, both physical and psychological, with a prevention-first focus. Stephanie has a busy private practice and runs gut and well-being programmes in collaboration with Goodwood Wellbeing in West Sussex. Stephanie sits on the advisory board of the Standards Authority for Touch in Cancer Care (SATCC) and is a willing and enthusiastic public speaker for professional and lay-audiences.

Previous works
'Why Eating Less & Exercising More Makes You Fat' (2016)
Explaining the 4 fundamentals to true health and vitality, questioning the received wisdom of the medical world.

Upcoming works
'Eat Your Body Lean'
A practical guide to achieving and maintaining a strong and vital body at any age.

Preface

I've been working in human health since the early 1990s: from physical therapies to psychotherapy to nutritional therapy, the practice of healing through food. Even so, not once, in over 3 decades of extensive and ongoing professional training, has the integral interconnectedness of physical well-being with mental and emotional regulation been a subject of study. Yet in my practice, in approaching mental health issues with the same whole-body, natural health philosophy I have used for decades in my work with physical health conditions such as type 2 diabetes, obesity, chronic fatigue, auto-immunity and more, I have seen first-hand how a healthy lifestyle approach allows the brain to become fitter and healthier, just as the body does. A healthier brain is more functional, more balanced and more resilient.

A few years ago however, the new discipline of nutritional psychiatry, the study of nutrition as medicine for the brain, began to produce solid science on the fascinating, intricate communication networks that integrate and influence every single part of the body, including the brain. Complicated systems such as digestion, immune function, hormone and metabolic status are no longer viewed as separate to one's mental health. The whole body works tirelessly as one united front to keep all the parts of us functioning in unison. As with physical ailments, for those with mental health problems the balance is off kilter, but maybe we've been looking in the wrong place for the reason why.

The gut (our digestive system) and the workings of the brain have a profoundly complex and co-dependent relationship. What is going on in one *will* be affecting the other. The brain can often feel indistinct, mysterious and 'other' than the body in many ways, whereas the gut seems far more accessible and more easily influenced through our food and lifestyle choices. Yet the brain and the gut share the same types of nerve cells and in many cases require and make the same nutrients and biochemicals and respond to many of the same influences. Effective management of mental health conditions, whether mild or severe, needs to take an integrative, whole-body approach, paying keen attention to digestion and diet. Good management of our mental health involves the wellness of our whole body.

The brain is not a self-contained unit and the highly complex regulation of its function does not all happen solely in the brain.

I write this book in the hope that it will help you think differently about what it means to have a mental health condition, whether your own or for those around you. We will explore why digestive health is fundamental to a happy brain, the role diet and lifestyle play on the gut microbes and how that can positively or negatively affect many aspects of brain function.

The great news is that we have considerable agency over our gut microbes through what we choose to eat and not eat. This makes the untouchable touchable: we can affect our brain and we can do it through our food. The worrisome, intimidating world of poor mental health comes right back to basics – what is on our plate.

A note to the reader

I began researching and writing this book in late 2020, during the Covid-19 pandemic. The world was locked down and, for obvious reasons, levels of anxiety and depression were skyrocketing, making this book more important than ever. However, the last few years have seen a huge flurry of research on the gut, the brain and mental health, requiring many updates and revisions. Inevitably, the book became longer and denser with each new research paper I read. When I finished the first draft it was too complex and not the accessible, user-friendly guide I intended to write. Several lengthy and technical chapters had to be cut out. The version you are reading today focuses on simple, practical ideas for how to *Eat Your Brain Happy* with some carefully selected theory to make clear the imperative of a healthy lifestyle for a happy brain.

If you would like to read the chapters I cut out, go to www.health-in-hand.com, where you will find a free PDF of this additional work, which may be more appropriate for those working in the field of mental health and well-being. This supplementary material provides a deeper explanation of the cellular signalling systems of the gut and the brain and should be read after finishing this book.

Introduction

It is a biological fact that the brain cannot function without a constant supply of nutrients and other compounds that are made in the gut and then transported up to the brain. So our brain is dependent on our gut functioning well. And what's the biggest influence on gut function? Food!

If you absolutely knew your depression or anxiety would improve, at least to some degree, with a change of diet, would you make those changes? Many people would consider this a nonsense question because it seems so implausible that something as truly awful as depression or cripplingly exhausting as anxiety could possibly be improved through something as basic as a change in what we eat. And yet, most of us know how too much caffeine, sugar or alcohol can change how we feel, think and function, so surely it's not such a stretch that our mental health might also be affected by what we choose to consume.

We now know that what we eat not only fuels our physical activity and well-being, it also feeds and affects the colony of microbes that live in our digestive system, for better or worse. We also know that those gut microbes, known as our gut microbiome, have a direct influence on our brain chemistry and function, for better or worse. If our diet is poor, our digestive system will suffer, and if our digestion is poor, we shouldn't be surprised if our brain suffers in some way too. It's a two-way street: when the brain is out of kilter, our ability to digest our food can be affected. Whether it's bloating, fatigue, hardly ever pooping or pooping way too often, or whether it's chronic depression, anxiety or panic attacks, these symptoms often stem from the same root cause.

> 'Living a life that supports mental well-being looks a lot like living a life that supports physical well-being.' [1]

The health status of our gut microbes is intrinsically linked to our whole-body health, the brain included. Feed them well and they will fuel our brain well – this is the exciting and life-changing science of nutritional psychiatry. Thanks to the wonderful work of Felice Jacka, a professor of nutritional psychiatry at Deakin University in Australia and founder and president of the Society for Nutritional Psychiatry Research, the science behind the idea that what we eat changes the way our brain works has developed rapidly over the past few years. Jacka and her team at the Food and Mood Centre have published hundreds of peer-reviewed studies showing the objective and subjective benefits of a change in diet in people diagnosed with mood disorders including depression and anxiety. She comments:

> 'Many studies from a multitude of countries now show that a dietary pattern higher in added sugar and fats, and ultra-processed foods, is linked to more emotional and behavioural problems ... as well as mental health.' [2]

Eating good food ensures that the brain has the energy and nourishment it needs to get stuff done. If the brain isn't getting enough of the right kind of fuel it will be forced to put on the brakes and that can show up as any number of mental health conditions. Not only that, what we eat affects our thoughts, our resilience, our tolerance to pain, our tolerance to others, how we respond to medications, how we sleep, how we wake – it's all part of one huge and fascinating system that is governed by the staggering mass of microbes living inside us.

Think of your brain as the heroic, hardworking, tireless and intrepid mountaineer reaching the summit and getting all the glory. Now think about what it takes to get that mountaineer up to the summit: down at base camp are all the intelligence, all the provisions, all the guidance on when to go, when to rest, when to hold back. The support team are working around the clock surveilling the conditions and sending up intel for the climber to achieve their goal. This is your gut microbiome, constantly sensing, communicating and guiding the brain's function to reach peak potential. The brain, like the mountaineer, is doing a lot of the heavy lifting, but the management system is coming from the gut.

Remember, the human brain cannot function without nutrients and other compounds that come from our digestive system (our gut), which are passed up to our brain. Therefore, by definition, the ability of our brain to regulate our mood, mental health and cognition depends on what we are eating and how well our digestive system is functioning.

Good gut health = Good mental health

Although this is still a relatively new field of research, the gut–brain connection is a proven biological process that is now being considered in the management of and potential recovery from anxiety, depression and many other mental health challenges. You may know someone who has been challenged by mental health issues, or maybe you are the one who is struggling to work out why your thoughts, mood and zest for life have been ravaged by anxiety or depression. Maybe you are experiencing changes in your emotional regulation or battling a profound lack of motivation and loss of joy; maybe you are painfully aware of your decreased tolerance of others; maybe you feel like you have lost something of your former, 'better' self, while being crippled by dark thoughts and a relentless sense of foreboding. All these experiences can be deeply troubling and may make you think that you are damaged, unfixable, even unlovable. Whether it's continuous despairing thoughts, a profound numbing of all feelings or a persistent and nagging sense that something awful is about to happen, depression and anxiety are very real conditions that are becoming increasingly common. What many of these pervasive symptoms are signalling is not that you have something fundamentally wrong with your brain, but rather that your brain is not functioning optimally due to its needs not being met. The former implies broken hardware, the latter is a much more fixable issue of correcting the signals the brain is receiving.

When I first began to understand the incredible co-dependence of the gut and the brain, it allowed me to start thinking of the brain and the body as one whole and integrated organism where any number of life and health dynamics could be affecting how well the brain works just as much as the body. Anything from poor sleep to the stress and pain of a physical injury, from unresolved emotional trauma to digestive issues or nutritional deficiencies – all of these influence mental health. There is a continuous flow of cause–effect, body–brain, brain–body. The influence of the body on the brain, and more specifically of gut health on brain health, known as the gut–brain axis, is now being intensively studied, and we have a growing understanding of the direct interplay of gut function with many mental health issues. This is an excerpt from a 2020 article in the *Annals of Medicine*:

> *There is increasing evidence that the gut microbiome and microbial dysbiosis [loss of healthy gut microbes] contribute to some of the more prevalent mental health and neurocognitive disorders, such as depression, anxiety, obsessive-compulsive disorder (OCD), post-traumatic stress disorder (PTSD), schizophrenia, bipolar disorder, and dementia as well as the behavioural and psychological symptoms of dementia through the microbiota-gut-brain axis.* [3]

So the gut has a far-reaching role in brain function. What's going on in our brain is not happening in isolation to our body, nor to our environment, our food choices or our levels of stress, joy or physical challenge. If we are depressed or anxious, our brain is not broken, it's just not functioning optimally. This is an incredibly significant shift in the understanding and treatment of poor brain regulation that results in mental ill-health. Knowing this puts us in a position to proactively improve our current physical and mental health while also protecting our brain from future neurological damage. Now that's exciting!

About this book

Eat Your Brain Happy explains this emerging field of whole-body mental health support and provides a detailed guide to how to approach your mental wellness differently, using a wide range of simple yet scientifically supported techniques.

> *This book is a tool and a guide, it is not a treatment protocol. While it is designed to provide a support system to improve mental well-being safely for everyone, it is important to emphasise that anyone experiencing mental ill-health should seek or continue with professional support and not, under any circumstances, change or stop medication without medical supervision.*

I have tried to keep the jargon to a minimum and the science accessible and concise. For those already well versed in the spellbinding goings-on of the body, I have included some Geek Boxes to satisfy my need to go into some of the more intricate and fascinating detail of the body–brain dance. But the book works perfectly well without you ever going anywhere near this information. For those looking for a more technical deep dive, there is also a free PDF on my website (www.health-in-hand.com) that explains much more of the new science behind the metabolic approach to mental wellness.

Part One addresses the biological mechanisms of anxiety and depression. I strongly believe that having a sense of why we might not be thriving can offer enormous motivation and clarity around what can be done to better manage these conditions.

Part Two is where the action happens. Here you will find how-tos for eating, sleeping, supplementing, moving, breathing and generally living in a manner that targets the body and brain communication systems. These are safe, non-extreme suggestions that you can practise on a regular and long-term basis to give your body the best chance to heal and self-regulate.

Eat Your Brain Happy aims to cut through the noise of the diet wars and focuses instead on what is most likely to be truly helpful to promote mental and physical health, particularly for those experiencing anxiety or depression. Natural health interventions help our body to help itself, creating the best environment for biological balance and self-healing without knowing all of the hows or whys. The good news is that studies are consistently finding it is the small and familiar lifestyle choices we make day to day, over the long term, that have the greatest impact on our mental well-being.

Small things done consistently create lasting positive change.

Managing expectations

There is no magic bullet, although for some people a few surprisingly simple changes can bring about lasting change very quickly. With all the complexities of what makes us human, coupled with what makes us individuals, it may take a while to find the right mix for you. I'm not expecting you to try to take on all the recommendations in this book all at once – that is usually a guaranteed way to add to overwhelm or feelings of hopelessness and despair when you fail to achieve what you've committed to. You may be ready for a big change and be able mentally, physically and practically to take on a lot all at once. Or you may do better by simply changing one thing in your morning routine to start with. As the new change becomes normal and a habit, then you can come back and decide on a second change. There is no order, there is no time limit, there is no right or wrong. Everyone will prefer a different starting point and degree of engagement.

What is critical is to get going, to do something. Just one change is far better than no change at all. Just one change can inspire hope and belief that you can reset your body and brain to a happier, healthier you.

PART ONE
YOUR BRAIN IS NOT BROKEN

CHAPTER ONE
Why Is It So Hard to Be Happy?

This book offers an evidence-backed, whole-body approach to managing depression and anxiety. First, we need to be clear what we're talking about.

Anxiety is hardwired to kick in when our nervous system detects some danger. It is a warning sign that we're not safe and therefore protective measures are required, pronto! This is a vital self-preservation response. It's a good thing. Without it, we are a sitting duck right in harm's way with no motivation to get to safety – or at least that's the message our brain is sending to our body via our nervous system.

> *Our anxiety does not come from thinking about the future, but from wanting to control it.* [4]

During extreme and rare situations when there is an actual, imminent threat to life, high anxiety triggers a rapid and intense arousal of the stress hormones, driving a call to action that ensures we save ourselves from the danger. This fabulous survival mechanism makes a lot of sense from an evolutionary perspective where the chance of being killed by a wild animal, a rival tribesperson or a swarm of angry wasps was very high indeed. It is key to appreciate this.

The experience of anxiety is there for a reason. It's a necessary and effective response to a perceived threat.

Paradoxically, despite relatively few truly life-threatening situations facing most people in the modern world, anxiety levels are dramatically on the increase. The powerful biochemicals driving the anxious state are present whether or not there is a real threat. If our brain chemistry is triggering the anxiety response, we are fearful, no matter how safe and secure we might actually be. Living with this hypervigilant, anxious overresponse means we are unable to soothe, calm, heal, digest, sleep, restore, relax, have fun, connect with others and be at peace with ourselves.

Depression is associated with words and experiences such as hopelessness, a sense of sadness, apathy, loss of self, lack of motivation, loss of purpose and place in the world, lack of self-worth and self-care. Feeling low and overwhelmed by sadness is a normal and rational response to something adverse that is happening or has happened to us or someone we are close to. We can feel depressed by the state of the world, or by being repeatedly let down, failed or disappointed by others. This is circumstantial or situational depression and can be a healthy, appropriate state of being as part of the human experience.

Feeling blue and despondent about life is understandable in our challenging times. These moments tend to lighten and pass when something distracts us from our gloominess: a call to a friend, watching a comedy show or reading a good book. However, if symptoms persist for more than two weeks, with unremitting or increasing feelings of hopelessness, self-doubt and worthlessness, this is generally considered to be chronic depression. Clinical or chronic depression is pervasive and largely unrelenting. We cannot be cajoled to 'snap out of it'. Depression is heavy, deep and casts a darkness over everything, sapping the slightest of motivation and meaning out of all that used to excite and drive us, making the most basic functions hard to fulfil.

Classic symptoms of chronic depression are a lack of pleasure, especially from things that used to be pleasurable; feeling low with a lost sense of purpose or meaning in life; a change in appetite, often a lack of desire to eat, or a drive to eat highly processed and hyperpalatable foods since they can provide a momentary lift of mood. Circumstances can be the catalyst, but there are usually deeper underlying causes that prevent natural recovery after a short period of time.

What is often challenging for both patient and clinician is discerning whether the experience of depression is an appropriate response in the context of the patient's life or is due to brain malfunction, because the symptoms can be the same. The joy of a natural, whole-body approach to mental wellness is that it doesn't matter which it is. Whether life is causing you to feel deeply depressed or your brain is currently unable to allow you to feel happiness, there are upstream ways that can help by supporting your own systems of healing and restoring a happy brain.

Bringing back the balance

There is strong, emerging scientific evidence that much of what can knock the brain off kilter and result in varying degrees of mental health challenge stems from a multitude of biological, sociological and environmental factors. These create imbalances within the whole body and not necessarily an illness, disease or dysfunction in the brain. Rather, anxiety and depression could be a message that your brain is not getting nourished and regulated appropriately, be it nutritionally, emotionally or spiritually, due to things going on elsewhere in your body and in your life. Fix your body and lifestyle imbalances and the brain will be able to regulate and restore better function in myriad ways.

Known factors contributing to depression and anxiety

- Lack of essential nutrients: a highly processed, nutrient-poor diet fails to nourish and heal all parts of the body, including the brain.
- Poor gut health: the gut microbiome has a superhighway to the brain. If the gut microbiome is not thriving, nor can our mental and emotional health.
- Hormonal imbalance: stress, sex and thyroid hormones are all influencing our brain's ability to self-regulate and balance.
- Chronic inflammation: if we are exposed continuously to diet and lifestyle factors that trigger ongoing (chronic) inflammatory responses within our body, our brain could be inflamed too. An inflamed brain is an unhappy brain.
- Lack of natural daylight: not having early-morning daylight especially and getting too much artificial, blue-spectrum light (from screens and LED lights) at night disrupt wake and sleep cycles, which are strongly associated with all aspects of poor mental health.
- Too much technology: excessive time spent on screens can remove us from the simple pleasures of real life and overstimulate our drive for more addictive pleasure hits, while providing very little (if any) true happiness and connection. Human beings are innately pack animals – we thrive on connection.
- Lack of natural movement: sitting too much, especially indoors, is associated with a whole host of poor physical and mental health outcomes.
- Disconnection: from ourselves, from others, from our communities and from nature.

If your mental and emotional health challenges are due to tough life circumstances, such as the loss of a loved one, living in a threatening situation or feeling lost, then anxiety and/or depression is an appropriate, normal, even healthy response. Supporting yourself through these difficult times with good food and lifestyle practices may seem trivial considering what you are going through, yet it could prove invaluable in creating greater tolerance to help you endure your pain and regain balance more quickly. How we come through and recover from trauma and great hardship is as much about our physical stamina as it is our mental fortitude. Good physical health and good mental health are teammates, supporting each other.

> *Accumulating evidence provides support for the existence of direct relationships between nutrition, stress susceptibility, mental health and mental function throughout the lifespan.* [5]

A great example of this is the work of Julia Rucklidge, a professor of clinical psychology at the University of Canterbury in New Zealand. Following two major earthquakes in the country in 2010 and 2011 and the mosque shootings in 2019, Rucklidge and her team studied the recovery responses of those who had suffered these major traumatic events and were given basic vitamin and mineral supplements. The results were clear:

> *Those who took nutrient pills had a clinically and statistically significant reduction in anxiety and an improvement in their mood, compared to those who received other treatments or no treatment.* [6]

If the cause of your mental unwellness is evident, with a situation outside of your control clearly driving your symptoms of depression and/or anxiety, then there are small but powerful actions you can take to help buffer the impact of your situational struggles. When you are faced with adversity, your body needs more care than ever, yet it's so hard to achieve. Having a toolkit of lifestyle tweaks that can provide some resilience and damage limitation at a time when your physical, mental and emotional states need all the help they can get can makes an enormous difference to how you experience and recover from these depleting events. Few people learn these tools at an early enough age to integrate them into our subconscious responses. For most people, when life throws us difficult, uncomfortable or threatening challenges we are more likely to neglect our most basic needs of good nutrition, good sleep, staying active and connecting with others. Providing such a toolkit to help restore balance is what this book is all about.

What if there's no reason?

For the many people who are suffering with mental health symptoms where there is not an obvious external cause, the struggle can be worsened by the frustration at there being no apparent reason for feeling so overwhelmed by life that they're unable to cope. Their internal dialogue adds to their distress: 'How can I be depressed when I am so fortunate/lucky/blessed; have a loving family/great job/beautiful home/money in the bank – when there's nothing wrong?'

If you just can't understand why you're so 'off' when everything seems to be so good, it could be your brain doing exactly what it should in the face of a lack – a lack of a specific nutrient or nutrients; a lack of high-quality sleep; a lack of rest and recovery time in an unrelenting schedule; a lack of exercise; a lack of social and personal connection; a lack of purpose, joy and awe. None of these things is easily measurable, but all can be profoundly influential on how you experience the world. Maybe, just maybe, your bouts of depression, panic attacks, heart palpitations or persistent feelings of doom come from your brilliant brain sending out a signal for help, calling for balance.

Think back to when you were last really well. What happened to change that? If you have some sense of the chain of events in your life, your biology and the subsequent impact on your emotional and mental well-being, then you have a great starting place to make changes. I often hear things like 'I was going through a really stressful time' or 'I was run down and got sick, took antibiotics and then the anxiety started'. This is a huge clue to why your brain is now on high alert.

You might not have considered that your sugar cravings, bloated belly, irritable bowel syndrome, skin disorder, low energy, joint aches or poor immune function could be at the heart of your depression and anxiety, because no one has joined up the physiological and psychological dots for you. With so much focus on a singular paradigm – that depression, anxiety or feeling low and overwhelmed is due to a lack of the 'happy brain chemical' serotonin – the solution offered has only ever been medication or therapy based. What if this is only a tiny part of the equation? More than 50% of people with depression and anxiety are not getting any relief from medication and therapy, yet little else has been on offer. Now there is a positive new approach that appears to be beneficial for many people with mental health issues, irrespective of what label they carry. Now you can take action to provide what your body and brain need to self-correct even if the cause of your unhappy brain is a mystery to you. Let's take a look at how.

Anxiety: What is your body telling you?

As I explained at the beginning of this chapter, anxiety is there to alert us to danger and to prompt us to take action, whether that be to run away, fight for our life or stand stock still – otherwise known as the fight, flight or freeze response. This is a necessary primal survival instinct that is in no way bad or wrong in the appropriate circumstances.

Today there may indeed be circumstances that require all-out self-preservation or protection of loved ones, but for most people most of the time, their anxiety is not in response to such a threat nor proportionate. Yet the body continues to sound the high-alert, fight, flight or freeze alarm: a pounding heart, blood pressure rocketing creating tension throughout the body, screaming alarm bells in your head and an often sickening, whole-body sensation of dread. High levels of anxiety can make you feel like you're going to die.

The feeling of lack of safety is not the same as not being safe, but the lived experience is the same in the moment because the brain is sending the same message regardless.

So what is going on? Our modern-day fight, flight or freeze alerts still signal 'all is not well', 'you are not safe', 'action is required', but occur because of small but unrelenting hits of things like this:

- Not enough quality sleep
- Poor hydration
- Poor nutrition causing poor gut health and malnourishment
- Unaddressed allergies and food sensitivities
- Poor blood sugar control often due to highly processed foods
- Constant social media alerts challenging our sense of 'am I enough?'
- 24-hour news, most of which is miserable or concerning
- Ever-increasing exposure to wi-fi and mobile phone signals emitting an electromagnetic frequency that is not natural to the earth and our bodies [7, 8, 9]
- Man-made chemicals in our food, air, water, personal care products, furniture, cars and clothing
- Mould-based toxin exposure
- Environmental heavy metal exposure, in particular lead and mercury
- An undiagnosed latent virus

Stress is an ignorant state. It believes that everything is an emergency. Nothing is that important. [10]

Any of these and many other seemingly innocuous events could be leading to an exhaustive state of fearfulness and foreboding, alerting our nervous system and triggering anxiety. Then factor in the challenge of interpersonal relationships, bills to pay, to-do lists that never get shorter and deadlines that rarely get met. If we get stuck in a place where we are routinely thinking about what is not good or right, we are perpetually triggering and reenforcing the neural pathways that wire our brains to be anxious and overwhelmed.

> **Our stress triggers are so pervasive that they have become normal and unremarkable yet our biology is responding like it's life or death. If we can think ourselves into a state of anxiety, we can think ourselves happy too.**

Depression: Does it serve a purpose?

Many thousands of clinical trials and papers have been written exploring the causes of and treatments for depression, with the consensus, until recently, assigning poor brain chemistry regulation, specifically low levels of serotonin, as the culprit. This is a highly simplistic view of a complex mental health state. That is clearly explained on the Harvard Medical School website:

> *Many chemicals are involved, working both inside and outside nerve cells. There are millions, even billions, of chemical reactions that make up the dynamic system that is responsible for your mood, perceptions, and how you experience life.* [11]

The family of drugs known as SSRIs or selective serotonin reuptake inhibitors have been prescribed for decades to help patients with depression, their mode of action being to make higher levels of serotonin available in the brain. But their use does not address why serotonin levels are low in the first place, if that is indeed the cause. Levels and interactions of serotonin, along with the many other brain chemicals, are constantly increasing or decreasing, ebbing and flowing, depending on the information and inputs coming from inside and outside of us.

Addressing one single brain chemical may tweak the symptoms of depression, which can easily be construed as an improvement or even a resolution, but it can never confer lasting change if there are multiple actions at play. It's like trying to stop a leaky roof by plugging only one hole out of many. We need not only to fix all the holes but to reinforce the roof by renewing the weak, faulty parts. That is what can be done through a full-body reset of diet and lifestyle.

An article in the journal Social Science & Medicine questions our modern take on depression, a condition that has been observed and written about for over 2000 years:

> *Depression is often framed as a disease or dysfunctional syndrome, yet this framing has unintended negative consequences including increased stigma. Here, we consider an alternative messaging framework – that depression serves an adaptive function ... signalling a need for help ... and using rumination to reduce distraction from external factors to solve complex social problems ... [rather than] the idea that depression is a purposeless disease.*[12]

For those experiencing depression, this is important to consider: it can have a purpose, it's not always about something being wrong. When feeling depressed can be related to something hard, bad or sad that has happened, a lack of joy, purpose, drive and happiness can be seen as the mind taking time for reflection, for healing physical and emotional bruises, for bearing and then coming to terms with the pain of love lost or hopes dashed. This is a time for inner reflection, a functional withdrawing from the busyness of the world, to process emotional and existential pain until time allows some healing to occur. Eventually, hope becomes an option again and laughter comes more easily.

Self-care for the brain

It's evident that there is no single cause of depression or anxiety, and there is no one experience of it either. I feel strongly that this point needs to be communicated more if the standard of care is going to change. We have to accommodate the idea that poor mental health is a full-body phenomenon, a biological system that is unable to provide adequate inputs, not just a wonky brain mismanaging one or two of its chemicals. The difference is key. Put the wrong fuel in the car, the car doesn't work, right? It's the same principle. Whatever the cause, your body needs a multipronged approach of self-care. If you were physically exhausted from running a marathon, you'd take a few days or weeks to rest up, eat more, maybe get a massage and soak in a hot bath. But who teaches us the self-care of our brain?

Biology (how your body works) and psychology (how your mind works) are intimately entwined. This helps to explain how two people can experience the same terrible event yet their post-trauma experiences can be entirely opposite. One may use their devastating experience as a catalyst to make significant, positive changes in their life, helping them to thrive on the gratitude of being a survivor and being buoyed by the concept of 'what doesn't kill you makes you stronger'. Someone else, even from the same family, living through the same traumatising event can be left unable to move on, emotionally and mentally incapacitated, with a sense of having lost something of themselves. What determines these different outcomes appears to be the mental and physical status of the individual before the event happens. If your body has optimal nutritional reserves to support a robust immune system, healthy gut and balanced stress response, coupled with a resilient external emotional support system, your chances of a good outcome after a traumatic event are far greater than someone who was already depleted, alone and struggling to cope with life before the devastation happened.

In the following chapters I will dive into these many variables so that you can begin to identify which areas of your life might need some adjustments to better support your brain and allow you to thrive. But first, we need a brief biology lesson.

CHAPTER TWO
The Biology of an Unhappy Brain

Happiness is a body-wide process

There are some common factors that seem to be universal happiness promotors despite a huge variety of cultures. One strong commonality among happy, healthy communities, wherever they may be in the world, is that they all eat a mostly local, mostly wholesome diet comprising largely ancestral, natural foods. They are also outdoors and active a lot and they feel part of something bigger than their immediate family circle – they have a community and a sense of belonging. They are eating and living themselves happy!

The situation in much (although not all) of the developed world is very different. It is no coincidence that as rates of obesity, diabetes, heart disease and cancer increase year on year, so too do rates of depression and anxiety. Poor health is poor health, whether it shows up in the body or the brain.

Rarely is there one simple fix for our health challenges, especially when it comes to our mental well-being. It could be to do with where we live: a busy road nearby creating constant air and noise pollution, or nasty neighbours who keep us awake all night and complain to us all day. These are not things that can be easily fixed. It could be we have pain from an injury that wears us down, not just because living with pain is exhausting and miserable but also because daily pain medication can be disruptive to the digestion and challenging to liver function, which over time could mean we absorb fewer nutrients and eliminate toxins less well. The less nourishment of all kinds we have and the more toxins, the more likely we are to have an unhappy brain – this is body-wide thinking.

> *Mental suffering is co-produced by poverty, trauma, and excessive medication use. Patients' guts are as imbalanced as their moods. Single vertical treatments make them worse rather than better.* [13]

But who is looking at these whole-body connections in our Western model of specialised medicine? A psychiatrist looks at your brain chemistry, a gastroenterologist your digestion and a hepatologist your liver function, but these aren't separate entities functioning in isolation, they all influence each other. This point is made beautifully clear by Ye Ella Tian, the lead author of a study evaluating the physical and mental health of over 85,700 participants. Tian concludes:

> *Our new study shows that poor body health is a more pronounced manifestation of mental illness than poor brain health.* [14]

Read that again. A study of over 85,700 people concluded that 'poor body health is a more pronounced manifestation of mental illness than poor brain health'.

You are what you digest

So where do we start to get whole-body healthy? Let's begin with the digestive system.

> **An unhappy gut makes an unhappy brain**
>
> *During drug trials for anti-depressant medication, researchers have to first make their mice depressed to see if the drugs they are testing help. How do you make mice depressed? Quite simply, you feed them an inappropriate inflammatory diet, usually a dairy protein and seed oil blend, which is indigestible to mice. This causes digestive issues, followed by poor gut microbial health, resulting in inflammation in the brain. The mice get depressed and then the drugs can be tested. The food–gut–brain–depression link has been known about for a long time in laboratories, so why has it not been applied to human health?*

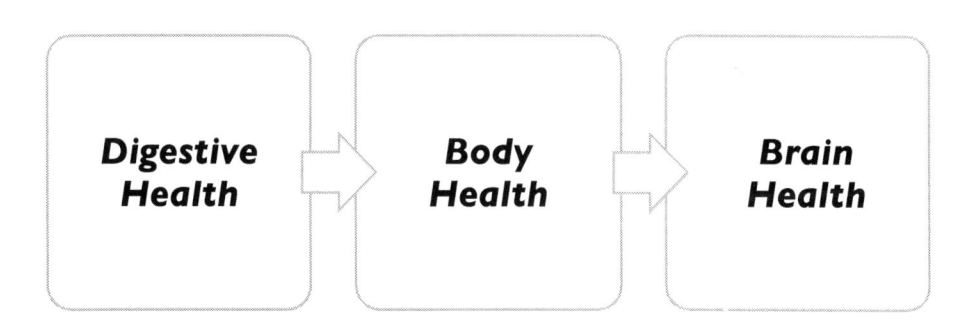

Digestive Health → **Body Health** → **Brain Health**

Poor digestive health can throw off the intricate management of our unique brain chemistry, resulting in pathways that release aggravating, depressive, anxiety-provoking or energy-suppressing chemicals instead of happy ones. If your diet or digestion is suboptimal, your brain can struggle due to a lack of the precursor ingredients required for optimal brain regulation that comes from good food and good digestion.

You are what you eat and digest.

> **Good mental health requires good digestion**
>
> *Our brain chemicals are made from amino acids. Amino acids are the end products of the digestion of protein coming from our food. This conversion of big chunks of protein into tiny, singular amino acids happens primarily in the stomach and upper intestines. When we swallow food, it passes down the throat into the stomach. The stomach prepares in advance to receive this food by producing high levels of very strong stomach acid, known as hydrochloric acid or HCl. This strong acid is absolutely integral to the brain getting the core ingredients to make happy brain chemicals.*

When we chew well, pay attention to our food, even smell what we're about to eat, the signal to make stomach acid kicks in. HCl then actions pepsin, a protein-digesting enzyme. Together they allow protein to become usable little units for the body and brain to mend our tissues and make our brain chemicals. This means good mental health is 100% dependent on good levels of stomach acid.

Eating quickly, while on the go, when stressed, in front of a screen, when driving or walking – all of these impair stomach acid production. This often leads to symptoms of indigestion such as burping, heaviness and fatigue after eating and eventually acid reflux or heartburn. The medications given for these symptoms further suppress the production of stomach acid. In the very short term that's probably OK, but think about what this might mean for our brain chemistry if our stomach acid is suppressed over the long term. No wonder studies have found use of acid-blocking medication to be a *'frequent cause of depression'*. [15]

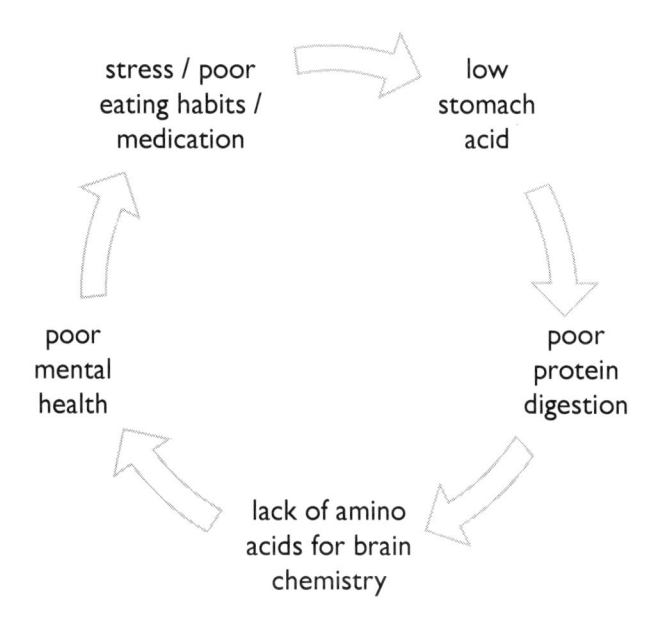

```
stress / poor              low
eating habits /          stomach
  medication                acid


                                              poor
     poor                                    protein
    mental                                  digestion
    health


              lack of amino
              acids for brain
                chemistry
```

If the core nutrients aren't in its fuel supply, our brain simply cannot make the chemistry and compounds required to run and balance its systems effectively – think low mood, poor memory, lack of motivation, feeling depressed and hopeless. If there is inflammation due to chronic high blood sugar or lack of quality sleep, or if there is an excess of stress hormones or an influx of inflammatory molecules coming from an unhappy gut, the brain cannot possibly get on with the nuts and bolts of healing and balancing – think headaches, migraine, anxiety, overwhelm, fear and dread. If our brain is fire-fighting, trying to protect itself from damaging toxins, chemical or mould exposure or lack of the healthy fats and proteins required for building and mending itself, then it is not going to be prioritising a happy balance of neurotransmitters and long-term brain function.

There is still so much to be understood about how the compounds in foods exert the power to balance and heal. But what is wonderful about using natural foods and lifestyle medicine to help us heal is that we don't need to know how it's happening nor exactly what the body or brain needs to course-correct. Provide it with a whole bunch of goodness and let your body decide what it wants and where that needs to go.

Small things done consistently can lead to exponential change.

Fuelling a happy brain

The brain is a very nutrient- and energy-hungry organ. Weighing only about 2% of our total body weight, averaging 3–4 lb (1.3–1.8 kg), it receives around 30% of the blood being pumped from the heart and consumes up to 25% of our daily calorie intake. That's a quarter of the calories we eat day to day being burned up by our busy brain – more than the liver and the heart and roughly equivalent to a 45-minute run. Activity requires energy and the brain never stops, so it's no wonder it's so ravenous, not just for energy (calories) but also for the nutrients in food like vitamins, minerals, healthy fats and proteins.

The brain is also the fattiest organ in the body, at about 60%, composed of various fats, including lots of cholesterol (this is a good and necessary part of a healthy brain) and lots of amino acids (which come from proteins in our food) – core ingredients to make brain chemicals. This provides a big clue to what we need to be eating to keep our brain happy and well fed: healthy fats and high-quality protein.

GEEK BOX

Cholesterol and a happy brain

The human brain contains more cholesterol than any other part of the body, about 20% of the total. Cholesterol is essential for healthy and happy brain functioning and low levels are associated with poor serotonin and dopamine management. Studies have found that very low levels can increase the risk of depression because cholesterol is integral to the nerve cell membranes that enable brain chemical signalling and brain cell receptors to function optimally.

Fat versus sugar (ketones versus glucose)

Management of the brain's dual fuel supply – sugar in the form of glucose and fatty compounds called ketones – is a key consideration. More on ketones later, but for now let's explore the impact of poor blood glucose management on mood and mental health.

As well as requiring adequate fat, protein and nutrients from the diet to make good-quality hardware, our brain also needs a steady supply of available fuel to allow the billions of neurons (brain cells) to fire constantly and consistently. What would happen if we were to stop eating for a while – where's the energy going to come from to keep our brain well fuelled? The sugar (glucose) in our blood is the first fuel to be used up. If we don't eat for a few hours it's normal for this blood glucose supply to run low. Blood glucose is like cash, quick and easy to use. The body then turns to a small store of glucose in the form of glycogen in the liver. This is like a current account, still giving us easy access to our funds. Once the liver glycogen starts getting low, as a smart dual-fuel machine the body turns to its long-term storage unit, our body fat. That's like a savings account, where the money is a little more difficult to get hold of but hopefully there's plenty of it!

In a metabolically healthy person, body fat is readily converted into energy when blood glucose and liver glycogen levels are low, but not zero. Burning of body fats kicks in before the glucose supplies are fully depleted. Keeping some stored liver glycogen and circulating blood glucose is important to fuel our small number of glucose-dependent cells and for any sudden, high-energy demands like running away from danger. Meanwhile, a healthy body happily runs on body fat until more food is consumed – this could be hours, or even days. Then when we eat some food, carbohydrates in particular, like bread, potatoes, grains, fruit and sugar, blood glucose levels increase, filling up the liver stores and providing fast fuel for the body and brain until the baseline is reached once more and fat burning kicks back in.

> **Our fuel reserves are stored as fat not sugar**
>
> *Roughly 5% of the body's energy is stored as sugar (glycogen), which leaves 95% of fuel reserves stored as fat.* [16] *Clearly the body is designed to run on fat rather than sugar!*

We have hundreds of thousands of calories of fuel stored in our body fat, some more than others, but even very slim people have at least a week's worth of ready-to-burn fat. This is how we survived famine when we lived off the land, so not eating for hours or days should be fine. But what if our fat cells aren't playing ball? What if we can't access all that stored fuel when there's no food coming in and our blood glucose hits baseline? It's like having a fridge full of food but the door is locked. This is what is happening to metabolically 'inflexible' people and it's why their hungry brain begins to struggle.

Metabolic inflexibility

Do you or someone you know get moody and short-tempered without frequent meals and snacks? Or maybe it's brain fog, word-blindness and poor concentration. Maybe it's increased anxiety and feeling more depressed. Poor blood glucose control can greatly disrupt an already unhappy brain, exacerbating symptoms far beyond simply influencing mood. If you notice your mental health symptoms worsening after a few hours of no calories from food or drink, this could be a sign of dysregulated blood glucose control, coupled with an inability to readily burn body fat for fuel. This is metabolic inflexibility, meaning poor management of your internal energy systems.

Metabolic inflexibility occurs for various reasons, largely lifestyle driven, and over time leads to a condition known as insulin resistance, a major root cause of a broken metabolic system (more on this to come). Insulin is a potent metabolic hormone essential to move glucose (coming from food) out of the blood into our cells, including brain cells, to provide quick fuel to be burned for energy production. If not immediately burned, a little can be stored in the liver and any surplus glucose is stored as fat. This critical process ensures that excess glucose does not stay in the bloodstream, as having high blood glucose for long periods is highly damaging, especially to the blood vessels and the brain. When we are metabolically healthy we are insulin sensitive, requiring only small amounts of insulin to keep blood glucose levels perfectly balanced and cells optimally fed, while allowing fat burning to kick in whenever blood glucose gets low.

> **Insulin is like a key to our cells, opening them up to allow glucose in for fuel. Good glucose management requires insulin-sensitive cells.**

However, a diet dominated by frequent meals and snacks of sweet and starchy foods – like sugar, brown or white bread and rice, milk chocolate, most highly processed foods (sugary liquids too) – greatly increases blood glucose levels way beyond the optimum. The body desperately tries to get glucose back to its safe level - around 1 teaspoon in the entire bloodstream, by triggering a surge of insulin to drive glucose out of the blood. A rapid spike in blood glucose triggers a large, rapid insulin response, often resulting in a mighty energy crash physically and mentally as blood glucose levels plummet. Critically, having high insulin levels also prevents fat cells being burned as fuel – the fully stocked fridge is padlocked. The result is no glucose or fat for fuel, which leaves our body and brain cells starved and very unhappy.

Eating sugary, starchy and highly processed foods is fine now and again. It's the daily hits of high blood glucose, triggering lots of insulin over and over again, that lead to poor glucose management and a mind-jarring crash. As we become less metabolically healthy and more metabolically inflexible, this response gets exaggerated. Smaller glucose spikes generate inappropriately large amounts of insulin, sending blood glucose plummeting below the lowest healthy level. Now we're hypoglycaemic (hypo = low, glycaemia = presence of glucose): hangry, irritable and easily overwhelmed. With low blood sugar comes an adrenaline rush as the body detects dangerously low levels of glucose and sends in the fight-or-flight hormones to bring levels back up. This adds to more stress, more instability, more disruption, more unhappiness in the brain.

Hypoglycaemia is commonly a cause of mid-afternoon concentration, mood and energy slumps, driving an often unconscious need for a caffeine and/or sugar/starch hit – think tea or coffee with biscuits, cake or chocolate. If lunch consisted of sandwiches, sushi (which often has added sugar), pizza, a burger and fries or a bunch of snack foods, the peak and crash of blood glucose will drive hunger a couple of hours later.

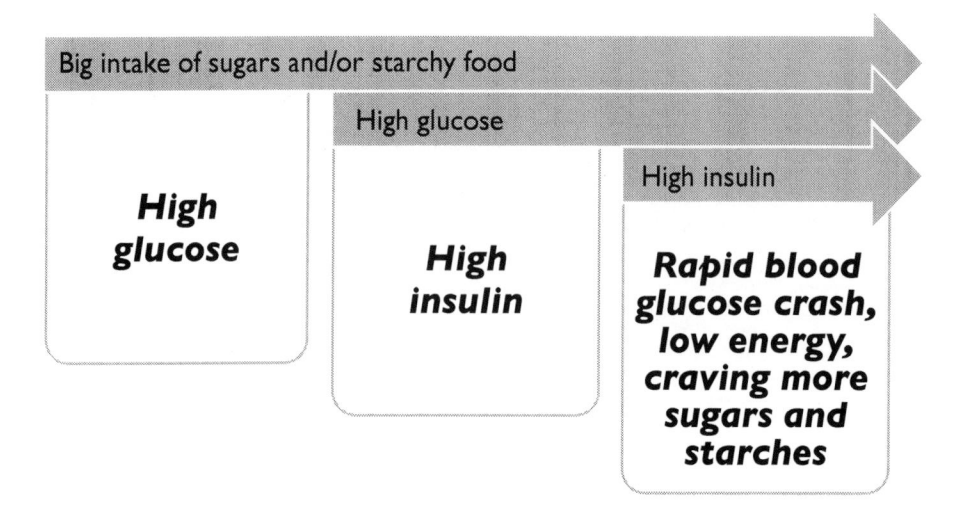

Big intake of sugars and/or starchy food		
	High glucose	
		High insulin
High glucose	**High insulin**	**Rapid blood glucose crash, low energy, craving more sugars and starches**

A huge number of people have this going on without knowing it. Eventually, over many years, it can result in insulin resistance, where cells 'resist' the influence of insulin, no longer allowing glucose inside the cell, leaving the glucose circulating in the blood despite high insulin levels. Over time, insulin resistance can become so bad that a person becomes a type 2 diabetes. However, well before there are signs of diabetes, people's bodies and brains are being deprived of sufficient fuel. This hiccup in both fuel supply systems – fat and sugar – forces the brain's function to be reduced, as it cannot possibly run at full throttle without a constant energy supply. Often this pre-diabetic, metabolically inflexible state first shows as bouts of anxiety, palpitations, feeling flushed and sweaty, unstable and lightheaded, along with sugar or carb cravings, low mood and an insatiable drive to eat coupled with a lack of satisfaction from food.

This constant drive to eat high-carb/sugary foods has further detrimental health effects like increased visceral fat storage – that's belly fat stored in and around the organs. Having more belly fat drives up inflammation, increasing stress hormones and further inhibiting fat burning, driving more sugar cravings and crashes, perpetuating this highly disruptive cycle.

> ***Poor blood glucose control due to insulin resistance is incredibly common and so often a factor in depressive and anxiety disorders.***

Many people wake in the early hours feeling anxious, hyper-alert and agitated for no apparent reason. But of course there is a reason: the brain is having a hypo! If dinner was disruptive to our blood glucose, with lots of bread, fries, pizza, pasta and pudding, and not enough healthy fat, protein and fibre-rich foods, blood glucose levels can peak and plummet at night, getting so low that the brain, which requires fuel to do its many functions while we sleep, has to activate the adrenal (stress) glands to drive blood glucose levels back up. This resolves the hypoglycaemia but results in an adrenaline rush that not only wakes us up, it leaves us with a racing mind and a feeling that all is not well. A broken night's sleep then drives hunger, sugar cravings and the need for quick fuel in the form of sugary and starchy foods, and so the roller coaster continues.

This is a physically and mentally exhausting scenario. Stress hormones, lots of insulin, high then low levels of sugar in the blood, broken sleep and anxiety all trigger inflammation, including in the brain. And the stress hormones triggered through this process end up being dumped in the gut, causing more inflammation and disruption to our digestion. Inflammation in the gut causes digestive upset and digestive upset causes an unhappy brain – see how it all ties together?

The insulin-resistant, 'diabetic' brain

Over a sustained period of time, likely decades, insulin resistance in the brain prevents proper energy uptake in the brain cells, creating a toxic soup of circulating blood glucose and insulin. High insulin and glucose in the brain lead to neuroinflammation. This is now being strongly associated with the development of Alzheimer's (often called type 3 diabetes) and other chronic, neurological progressive illnesses, including depression. With an estimated 88% of Americans suffering from insulin resistance [17] – and where the US goes the UK tends to follow – is it any wonder that depression is now the leading cause of disability worldwide?

> *a moderate increase in insulin resistance ... was linked to an 89% increase in the rate of new cases of major depressive disorder.* [18]

One study found that in certain patients having insulin resistance was stopping the brain using their psychiatric drugs. When bipolar patients were put on a diet with very few sugars and starches, insulin levels reduced, insulin sensitivity improved, and the patients' brains were then able to utilise their drugs. If insulin resistance can inhibit powerful drugs from working in the brain, what could it be doing to the use of the brain's own chemicals in patients with depression and anxiety?

> **Alzheimer's is increasingly being referred to as type 3 diabetes, diabetes of the brain. Many mental health issues are thought to have a similar origin.**

To avoid this happening, we need to be eating fewer of the foods that aggressively elevate blood glucose levels, and eating them less often, while employing some crafty health tricks to lessen the impact when we do (we'll look at those in Part Two). The foods that are helpful and not harmful for blood glucose control are also largely foods that support gut health and inflammation management – and that's no coincidence.

Why moving muscles matters

Eating sugary and starchy foods like rice, bread and potatoes is perfectly appropriate for people who eat and move, eat and move because the glucose that goes into their bloodstream after eating is immediately sent to their muscles to fuel the movement – this is how we are designed to function. If blood glucose is low and we need to move, our body fat fuels the movement instead – a simple, effective dual-fuel system. Our muscular system is by far the greatest sink for blood sugar disposal. Muscular contractions, even with gentle activity, rapidly draw blood sugar out of the bloodstream into the fibres of the muscles. Hence, the more muscle you have the more likely it is you will be metabolically fit and well. However, if we eat and sit, keep eating and keep sitting, the blood sugar levels rise and stay high resulting in a large insulin response to get the blood glucose back down to safe levels. Over time, insulin resistance occurs, where insulin becomes less good at moving the glucose from your blood, into your muscle cells, liver cells and brain cells, forcing your cells to reduce function. The resulting high blood glucose and high blood insulin can eventually lead to type 2 diabetes, but the brain can struggle with this 'diabetic' scenario long before your body does - remember, Alzheimer's disease is being termed by some experts as type 3 diabetes.

Metabolic psychiatry

Most of us are born with brains that are happy to run on either fat (ketones) or sugar (glucose). If there's glucose in the blood, the brain burns that glucose. When glucose is low, fat burning takes over and the brain runs on fat. As long as we remain metabolically flexible, meaning our blood glucose and insulin levels are well managed, the brain has the option of sugar or fat for fuel.

However, some people have brains that simply do not do well on glucose as a fuel source, despite their having good metabolic health. Rather than having dual-fuel brains they have single-fuel, fat-burning brains dependent on a constant supply of ketones. If their diets are high in sugars and starches, and/or they are metabolically inflexible, their fat-dependent brains will be starved of fuel on a fairly constant basis, driving mood and mental health mismanagement. This is the theory behind what is termed metabolic psychiatry.

All our brains love to run on ketones, which are fast-fuel clean brain-energy fat bombs, and many of us have brains that flip-flop between post-meal glucose and ketones when we're not eating, such as when we sleep, without us even noticing the switch. The more glucose we get from food the more the brain is running on glucose rather than ketones. But if we have a brain that wants only ketones for fuel, every time we eat something with sugars and starches the brain is being starved. Couple this with the common condition of metabolic inflexibility, meaning someone who doesn't readily burn body fat when they're not eating, and then the brain has neither glucose nor ketones for fuel. This leaves it very vulnerable to energy crashes and mental health disruption.

> *If your brain is running low on energy, your mental health will suffer.*

Metabolic psychiatry is acutely focused on ketones for mental health management. Increasing numbers of studies and clinical trials are finding that people with persistent and treatment-resistant mental health issues are responding exceptionally well to a diet that promotes the brain running on ketones in preference to glucose. Chris Palmer, assistant professor of psychiatry at Harvard Medical School and a practising psychiatrist, addresses mental illness as a metabolic issue in his book Brain Energy. This features many clinical examples of treatment-resistant patients making astounding progress when their brains started to run on ketones achieved through a change in diet.

It appears some people are genetically predisposed to having brains that fare far better on ketones rather than glucose. [19]

To shift your body from being a poor fat burner to becoming an efficient fat-burning machine, management of your blood glucose system is essential. This can be achieved through changing your diet and further finessed through adopting other nutrition and lifestyle strategies, all outlined in Part Two. Remember, you may have no sign whatsoever that your mental health struggles are down to a lack of ketones. You can appear to be physically fit and well, but that doesn't mean your brain is. By adopting a diet that allows ketones to be your primary brain fuel, you might discover that your anxiety or depression is down to an energy crisis. Surely it's worth finding out.

GEEK BOX

Ketones: Brain-friendly super-fuel

It has been known since the 1920s that a high fat, very low-carb diet, a ketogenic diet, greatly improves severity and frequency of seizures in children and adults [20] *whose epilepsy does not respond to medication. This medical dietary intervention has been approved for decades with the understanding that this way of eating mimics fasting, triggering ketone production, greatly benefitting patients with seizure-prone brains. This theory is now being applied to people struggling with treatment resistant* mental health conditions. This makes sense when we consider that many modern lifestyle factors such as our food choices, eating frequency and stress levels, prevent natural ketone-production occurring, helping to explain, at least in part, the exponential rise in mental health diagnoses. For those people whose brains do not function well on glucose as their main fuel source, as with patients with drug-resistant epilepsy, shifting towards a more ketogenic diet could provide great benefit. If your brain is a happy fat burner, preferring ketones over glucose for fuel, but is deprived of ketones due to excess blood glucose, turning off fat burning and therefore ketone production, it's inevitable that your brain is going to struggle.

Ketones are a clean and highly efficient energy source, not only for the brain but for almost every cell in the body. The big determining factor here is that we can only produce ketones when our insulin and blood glucose levels are low enough. As soon as we eat sugars and starches, insulin is produced and body fat burning is turned off. While there is quick fuel in the form of sugar (glucose) in the blood, we run off that. Once our blood glucose gets low, the liver tops up that blood glucose using its small store of sugar, called glycogen. Once that starts to run low, the liver converts body fat into ketones. We have a vast fuel source, our body fat, to keep us going through famine or long hunts, whatever might have prevented us from eating for long periods in ancient times. With our modern diet of relatively continuous sugar and starch, many people, much of the time, never create the opportunity for fat burning and therefore ketone production. That's fine if we have ideal body fat, very good blood glucose control and a brain that's happy to run on glucose alone, but that's rarely the case.

This is all readily reversible with a change in diet. The trouble is that the body gets out of the habit of fat burning and it can take some training to get it back up to speed to be able to quickly and effortlessly create ketones in the face of low glucose. Over time, with a reduction in sugars and starches, gradually prolonging your overnight fast to 12 hours or longer, and exercising appropriately, you can become a metabolically fitter, fat-burning ketone maker and see how your brain responds. See Part Two for more on this.

> **The evidence is compelling**
>
> *Albert Danon, a psychiatrist who works with patients who have severe and persistent mental health issues, such as major depressive disorder, bipolar disorder and schizophrenia, that do not respond to medication, conducted a small but significant study in France. He took 31 adults from his patient group, working with them in a hospital setting to ensure adherence to the plan, and changed one thing only – their diet. The protocol was quite extreme, a very low-carbohydrate meal plan known as the ketogenic diet for up to 248 days. This low-sugar, low-starch diet works very effectively at rapidly reducing levels of glucose in the blood. The outcomes were extraordinary: 100% patients had improvement in symptoms; 43% achieved clinical remission; 64% were discharged on less medication; 96% lost weight.*

A quote from Dr Danon says it all:

> *[we saw] significant and substantial improvements in depression and psychosis symptoms and multiple markers of metabolic health … weight, blood pressure, blood glucose and triglycerides.* [21]

The fact that almost all of these patients lost weight is not a happy coincidence nor insignificant. Loss of body fat reduced inflammation around the body, which then helped the patients regain better metabolic function, stimulating a whole-body shift from sluggish and 'grumpy' metabolic health to a better, self-regulating body and brain. One of the key improvements from these dietary changes was better insulin control or, more specifically, regaining insulin sensitivity – the reversal of insulin resistance. With insulin sensitivity comes improved blood glucose control and the ability to readily burn body fat again, hence the fat loss. Added benefits were reduced triglycerides (bad fats in the blood) and lower blood pressure. All of these improvements led to a reduction in inflammation around the body and brain, which then facilitated a more balanced and healing environment through the whole body, including the brain.

Critically, by becoming metabolically flexible, reducing blood glucose and reversing insulin resistance through a low-carbohydrate diet, these patients were able to burn body fat to make ketones to fuel their brains, and as a result massively improved their mental health.

Another study put 262 outpatients with type 2 diabetes along with mild clinical depression on a low-carbohydrate diet for 10 weeks. More than half no longer met the medical criteria for depression after this period.[22] Diabetes is a metabolic disorder. These people may have been depressed because they had diabetes, but what we are seeing from these studies is that a change in diet that improves metabolic health also improves mental health.

A pilot trial put patients with both metabolic and severe, medicated mental health issues on a ketogenic diet for four months. The clinical lead Dr Sethi, founder of the metabolic psychiatry clinic at Stanford Medicine, reported quotes from participants, one of whom stated:

> *Since being on the diet, I haven't noticed any significant anxiety level or attacks. And I've been able to work through basically everything I've come across.* [23]

These are exciting examples of how far-reaching and literally life-changing a different diet can be. Metabolic issues such as insulin resistance, commonly seen in individuals with mental health issues, are clearly impeding good, robust mental health and well-being.

With so much known about how to very effectively, quickly and safely reverse metabolic issues through changes to diet and lifestyle, there is a persuasive

argument emerging to make this a starting strategy for mental wellness, not a last resort.

With improvements in insulin resistance, body fat begins to reduce, especially the visceral fat inside and around our organs, which skinny people can be carrying as well as those who are overweight. As visceral fat reduces inflammation goes down, and fatty deposits in the liver and pancreas are reduced and eventually disappear, allowing ketone production and insulin sensitivity to improve. Regain insulin function and hey presto, energy levels improve and healing, both physical and mental, kicks in. This results in people feeling better on so many levels, whether or not insulin resistance was part of their mental health condition. When we feel physically well, managing mental ill-health gets easier.

> **Important note:** *The degree to which someone has to reduce sugar and starch intake to reverse insulin resistance is not nearly as extreme as carbohydrate restriction for consistent ketone production as in the medical trials described above. Simply avoiding refined sugars and carbs (as explained in Part Two), reducing sweet fruits and not snacking are often sufficient to achieve improvements in metabolic flexibility (insulin sensitivity), which may be enough to keep your brain happy. For those who have ketone-dependent brains, more extreme restriction of carbohydrates and higher healthy fat intake may be required to initiate adequate ketone production for a happy brain, but again, it may not be necessary to be in full ketosis all of the time to experience significant benefits. If, after following the recommendations in Part Two, you find only limited benefit, it may be you need the more extreme end of a low-carb diet, in which case it is important you seek professional help to move to an appropriate ketogenic diet safely.*

Taking in the sunshine

Another hormone important to the brain is vitamin D. This is actually a pre-hormone and a hugely important signalling molecule connecting many systems throughout the body and brain.

If you are low in vitamin D, everything in your life is likely to feel much, much harder.

Vitamin D is known as the sunshine vitamin because you can make it through skin exposure to the sun. If you live in a country with limited sunshine or if you keep covered or limit your exposure to the sun for religious or other reasons, you are not going to be making much, if any, vitamin D from being outdoors. Food sources are limited and if you are stressed and depressed you are likely to have compromised digestive function, which could be impairing your ability to absorb the little vitamin D that makes it into your diet.

Every cell in the brain has a receptor for vitamin D and it has been known for decades that vitamin D deficiency is associated with poor mental health. The vast majority of people in the UK and much of the northern hemisphere are vitamin D deficient, yet GPs are reluctant to test; even if they do, you are told you're fine as long as your levels aren't in the highly deficient range where you're at risk of getting rickets!

Achieving ideal levels of vitamin D often requires a concerted, very proactive approach, which we will explore in Part Two. This is just one quick example of one of the very many vitamins, minerals and other nutrients our hungry brain needs to be fully functional, adaptable and happy.

Styling your life

Hopefully you are beginning to get a sense of how our thoughts, feelings and the way we experience our world are intimately joined up with what we eat and also how we live. Our body needs a balanced and healthy lifestyle to function well. Too little exercise, too little sleep, too little joy or too much stress and it starts to show signs of being out of balance and unwell: low energy, weight gain, joint pain and high blood pressure. Most people will accept that a metabolic condition like obesity, heart disease or type 2 diabetes is a logical outcome of leading a consistently unhealthy life. But what if our brain is just as vulnerable, if not more so, to our lifestyle choices? What if our brain's ability to stay fit and well, to be resilient to stress and keep 100+ neurochemicals in balance, is also hugely determined by what we do and don't eat, how we sleep, our stress levels and the quality of the air we breathe and the water we drink?

Lifestyle interventions are gradually but increasingly being considered as an essential initial approach to mental health problems, rather than relying on medication. Having a mental health issue that requires support and specialist care is no different to having a broken bone and needing to avoid certain types of physical activity while getting physiotherapy for the fracture to heal. Yet we tend to consider these two health challenges very differently. If we accept that both scenarios are a sign of imbalance due to too much stress on a system of the body, be it excess impact on a bone causing it to break or lack of essential nourishment of all kinds for the brain causing a disruption in brain chemistry, then we can start to approach mental health recovery without stigma and with a great deal of hope and personal agency.

> ***Your physical health affects your thoughts, and your thoughts affect your physical health.***

There is much more on exercise, sleep and managing stress in Part Two. For now, I've mentioned inflammation several times in this chapter, so let's take a deep dive into what that means.

CHAPTER THREE
Inflammation

Inflammation is a mechanism of the body that is essential to keeping us alive. When we cut our finger open, sprain an ankle or come into contact with a nasty infectious bug, we want our immune system to launch an acute inflammatory response to kill off the bugs or heal the cut or sprain. A high temperature and sweaty brow, a red, scabby wound or a swollen, hot joint – all of these are signs of the body healing itself through an amazingly complex, innate, life-saving defence response.

This integral part of our immune system is something that evolved over millennia to help us survive the challenges of a hunter-gatherer lifestyle with all the attendant risks of injury and attack. As we came down from the trees and started walking the earth in our bare feet, allowing all manner of parasites, bacteria, viruses and more to pass into our bloodstream through the mouth and the skin via cuts and grazes, it learnt, adjusted and influenced our genetics to pass on its invaluable immune education to the next generations. This exquisitely smart defensive response is found only in vertebrates and goes a long way to explaining how we exist today at the top of the food chain.

Hence the acute inflammation triggered by our immune system is absolutely one we need to have working well but, like all our bodily systems, it's about balance: too much or too little immune response and we can be in trouble.

As with stress, inflammation becomes problematic when it's chronic – ongoing, unrelenting, inappropriate. The causes of chronic inflammation are many and complex. It's essential to appreciate that while inflammatory responses are being triggered the body is unable to heal, repair, restore and balance itself. While acute inflammation is protective, chronic inflammation is damaging, putting the brakes on digestion, healing and the critical gut–brain communications that help keep us balanced, happy and healthy.

Does an inflamed body cause an unhappy brain?

Researchers have not only found evidence of increased inflammatory markers in those who are depressed compared to those who are not, but also an association between systemic (body-wide) inflammation and further emotional dysregulation in the form of fearfulness (anxiety), being bothered by things (anxiety), hopelessness about the future (depression) and feeling like a failure (depression). The researchers described the link:

> *Anxiety is a signal of danger, perceived fear and threat. If this is an on-going situation it becomes a state of chronic stress. Chronic stress creates systemic (body and brain-wide) inflammation. Inflammation is associated with depressive disorders.* [24]

In conventional psychiatry mental imbalances are still very much considered an 'inside the brain' issue, without much regard being paid to what the rest of the body is doing. This is because, up until very recently, it was accepted that the body could not affect the brain directly due to the highly selective and protective nature of the blood–brain barrier blocking entry to anything damaging.

However, over the past 10 years it has become evident that this is not the case. Both the lining of the gut, a tightly controlled membrane that selectively allows nutrients to pass from the gut to the bloodstream, and the blood–brain barrier, which only allows into the brain what is absolutely necessary, can become overly permeable or 'leaky'. Large and inappropriate substances can pass from the gut into the bloodstream, causing the immune system to go haywire and leading to subsequent errant inflammatory responses. That results in the blood–brain barrier also becoming leaky, allowing the misplaced inflammatory compounds in the blood to pass into the brain. This causes the brain to become inflamed, potentially leading to mood and mental health disruption. Caroline Ménard, assistant professor of psychiatry and neuroscience at Université Laval and CERVO Brain Research, explained:

> eventually, you will have some tiny holes in the blood-brain barrier of the brain. And this will allow inflammation to pass from the blood into the brain, and this will eventually change the neurons and all the cells that create behavior and who we are. [25]

We are all susceptible to leaky membranes. It could be due to a course of antibiotics or having a gut that is sensitive to wheat or gluten. A high-sugar diet or one high in emulsifiers (chemicals used in packaged foods for texture and shelf-life) and other man-made chemicals in processed foods could be a cause, as could excess alcohol, chronic stress or even too much exercise. All of these have the potential to activate a leaky gut and a leaky brain. However, there is one culprit recently identified as a major trigger for the leakiness of both these protective barriers and as a super-inflamer if it gets into the bloodstream: lipopolysaccharides (LPS).

LPS are a toxic waste product produced when not-so-good gut bacteria die off. Gut bacteria of all kinds are continually reproducing and dying off and are ordinarily harmlessly eliminated via our poop. But if certain bacteria overgrow due to an unhealthy, unhappy gut, they release toxins, LPS, which build up, causing a leaky gut. The LPS then 'leak' into the blood where their very presence is now thought to be one of the most aggressive inflammatory triggers around the body and in the brain. The inflammation they cause triggers a major stress response. Then excess stress hormones in the gut cause more leaky gut, hence more LPS leaking into the blood and brain – a two-way perpetual cycle causing damage and reducing healing in the body and brain.

The title of a review article published in 2022, sums this up perfectly:

> *Gut Imbalance Imbalances the Brain: A review of gut microbiota association with neurological and psychiatric disorders* [26]

With such a direct connection between gut health and brain health, living in a gut-friendly way – one that reduces inflammation – is clearly an imperative for our mental wellness.

GEEK BOX

**Lipopolysaccharides –
an inflammatory monster molecule**

LPS come from the natural cycle of a type of bacteria know as gram-negative bacteria. When these bacteria dye off in the colon they shed an outer coat, which is known as an endotoxin. This bacterial waste product should be passed out in the stool with no ill effect. However, if instead the LPS enter the blood due to a leaky gut, the immune system is triggered and a mass of inflammatory reactions occur. LPS are one of the most common reasons for systemic inflammation in the Western world as modern dietary and lifestyle habits cause damage to the gut lining, allowing these endotoxins (toxins made inside the body) to pass into the bloodstream. LPS in the bloodstream trigger an inflammatory response through the production of interleukin 6, an inflammatory cytokine (cell-signalling molecule) that has been shown to cause the protective barrier of the brain to become leaky. This leads to debris that should not be able to reach the brain passing across the blood–brain barrier, generating neuroinflammation, which is disruptive to a happy brain balance. LPS also disrupt neurotransmitter balance, as they interfere with the binding of serotonin and dopamine to receptors in the brain and decrease production of these 'feel-good' chemicals together with GABA and melatonin, while increasing levels of the agitating, disruptive brain chemical glutamate. This can be experienced symptomatically in numerous ways, but commonly as depression and anxiety. For more on the science behind inflammation, go to the PDF on my website: www.health-in-hand.co.uk.

> **An anti-inflammatory effect**
>
> *As the chemical imbalance theory of depression continues to be challenged due to lack of evidence that depressed patients have low serotonin levels, one explanation for why antidepressants do appear to have a benefit for some people is that they have an anti-inflammatory effect (rather than a serotonin effect).[27] New anti-depressant medications are being developed for drug-resistant depression and anxiety that specifically address inflammation in the brain by blocking inflammatory cytokines.*

Managing your inflammation is managing your mental health

Good gut health, careful blood glucose management and reducing your level of stress – living a life that heals more and inflames less – is fundamental to a happy brain. In Part Two you will find many ways to correct leaky gut and brain barriers while nourishing your gut microbes. Meanwhile, look through the following lists of anti-inflammatory practices to see if there are a few changes you can start to make today to decrease your inflammatory triggers.

Pick one or two from these lists that you feel you can get going on straight away, to start the shift towards a less inflaming way of life.

Anti-inflammatory practices 101

For your body

- Buy organic food where possible. When you have to be selective, use EWG's Dirty Dozen™ (https://www.ewg.org/foodnews/dirty-dozen.php) and Clean Fifteen™ (https://www.ewg.org/foodnews/clean-fifteen.php) to prioritise which foods to buy organic.

- Reduce the amount of packaged/highly processed foods you eat – the fewer ingredients, the better.
- Try cutting out wheat for a couple of weeks to see if you feel better.
- Eat well at mealtimes and try not to snack. Periods of not eating help reduce blood glucose levels, which reduces inflammation.
- Aim for at least four days a week alcohol free, but don't be tempted to binge drink on the days you are having alcohol.
- Check food labels for artificial sweeteners. No one needs them and they upset your insulin response, your gut microbes and your mitochondria (cells that make energy).
- Get a water filter for all your cooking and drinking needs. A good jug filter is a great start to help reduce your chemical intake from the water supply, especially chlorine, a bleaching agent, which can be detrimental to good gut microbes. Make sure you change the filter regularly.
- If you're exercising daily, consider doing less, especially if you're feeling constantly fatigued, achy and irritable and/or if you are addicted to exercising – a big warning sign.
- Use non-scented, non-foaming personal care products and a natural deodorant rather than a chemical-based antiperspirant. The skin absorbs the chemicals you put on it.
- If you wear makeup, look for mineral-based, non-scented, natural, organic brands.

For your brain

- Sleep – work on your attention to detail around the timing, environment and quality of your sleep. Part Two has a whole section on this.
- Practise some form of meditation, journaling or calming breathing practice daily.

- Breathe through your nose, even when exercising and certainly when sleeping if you can.
- Move more, sit less. Try three-minute bouts of 'exercise snacking'.
- Always leave at least 12 hours from your last calories to your first calories the following day.
- Be conscientious about having daily doses of brain-protective nutrients and foods (more about this in Part Two).
- Manage any toxic thoughts – your thinking has a direct effect on your biology.

For your home

- Stop using artificial air fresheners and artificially scented household sprays and candles. The scents are made from man-made chemicals that give off VOCs, volatile organic compounds known to have various poor health implications [28] – breathing in chemicals can be inflammatory.
- Clean your house with natural agents like white vinegar, lemon juice and bicarbonate of soda or use more ecological brands.
- Use eco laundry balls instead of detergent – it's better for you, your clothes and the environment.
- Ventilate your home and workspace better to avoid chemicals accumulating in the air. You might want to consider getting a HEPA air filter for your/your children's bedrooms.
- Get lots of houseplants – they're great air cleaners, especially peace lilies, spider plants, palms and ferns, and they help to ease anxiety.
- Put a chlorine filter on your shower feed – it's easy, cheap and highly effective at reducing the amount of chlorine entering your body through the skin.

CHAPTER FOUR
Which Is in Charge, Your Gut or Your Brain?

There is an organ within the gut that has been largely ignored until very recently. It is a complex organism collectively termed the gut microbiome. Vast numbers of microbes, in their tens of trillions, are increasingly being understood to be fundamental to our physical and mental well-being, influencing the way our brain and body function and heal through their regulation of cellular nourishment, the immune and inflammatory system, hormonal balance, brain chemistry and so much more.

The gut–brain dynamic

There are, on average, ten times more microbes living in your gut than you have human cells, with the whole gut microbiome weighing around 3–4 lb (1.5–2 kg). The numbers are almost beyond comprehension, but estimates put the figure at around 80 trillion gut microbes – that's more stars than there are in the Milky Way!

Having large numbers of these microbes is important, but so too is their diversity. Experts on the microbiome widely accept that having a wide range of commensal (beneficial) microbes in the gut is a marker of good health. When the gut microbes of people who still live wild, hunter-gatherer, ancestral (and grubby) lives are analysed, there is far more diversity than for someone living an inner-city, typical Western life. What is being lost is not clear. The exact strains of bacteria, fungi, parasites, archaea and viruses that all come together to form an individual's microbiome are so complex and bespoke that there is no way of knowing what someone may have lost due to ongoing antibiotic treatment or a diet high in sugars and man-made chemicals, which may have killed off certain strains to the point where they are no longer present. How can you know what you've lost if you don't know what was there in the first place?

John Cryan, a microbiome researcher at University College, Cork, ran experiments on mice to see how their behaviour changed when their good gut bugs were eliminated. He noted that the germ-free mice (meaning they have no gut microbes) *'act in ways that mimic human anxiety, depression and autism'*. [29]

This ancient system of microbial cells and human cells supporting each other has evolved over millennia. The microbes that live in us and on us existed well before we did. They likely came from ancient soil and took up residency within us to be provided with a regular supply of fuel from the food we eat, and in return they help keep us healthy. If we don't reinstate some basic principles of ancestral living, this microbial eco-system is vulnerable to significant harm. That doesn't mean shunning progress, but it does mean maintaining and prioritising certain ways of eating and living that our body, microbiome and brain will recognise as good and hence allow us to flourish.

Although the majority of the human microbiome is found in the large intestine (or colon) and lower sections of the small intestine, we also have microbiome colonies throughout the body. The second largest colony of microbes lives in our mouth – the oral microbiome. Beneficial microbial colonies are also found on the skin, up the nose, in the liver, in the mucus lining of the lungs, in the vaginal canal and even in breast tissue. The gut microbes connect with all the other microbiomes in the body, allowing for whole-body cross-talk. In so doing, they can manage our immune, inflammatory and healing responses appropriately.

These different biomes comprise hugely differing types of microbes, with skin and gut microbes being as far removed from each other as the microbes that live in the desert are from those at the bottom of the ocean. Yet these diverse colonies communicate with each other to organise responses to environmental and biological triggers.

> **Oral hygiene**
>
> *If we have poor oral hygiene, nasty bugs can be thriving in our saliva and around our teeth and gums. We swallow anywhere from 500 to 900 times a day, so if our saliva has unhealthy microbes in it, they are passing into our digestive system, which can negatively affect our gut microbes. Unhealthy oral microbes can also pass up into the brain, causing mental and neurological health issues. A standard mouthwash is not the answer – it's like an antibiotic, killing both the good and the bad. Encourage a healthy oral microbiome through a good diet, staying well hydrated, keeping your mouth closed when breathing and trying to kick cigarettes and vapes.*

Until very recently it was thought that the brain was sterile, but now microbes are being discovered within brain tissues too. As with all the microbial colonies around the body, there can be good brain microbes keeping the system running smoothly, and there can be pathogenic, damaging bugs causing trouble. Bad gut bugs can lead to poor digestive function and digestive disruption. Bad bugs in the brain lead to poor brain function and brain disruption. Brain disruption can lead to the brain's energy systems falling short and this can result in mental health disorders:

> *Dysbiosis, an imbalance or alteration in the composition of the brain microbiota, has been associated with several neurological and neuropsychiatric disorders, including AD [Alzheimer's], multiple sclerosis, Parkinson's disease, depression, and anxiety.* [30]

Given the intrinsic connection the gut and the brain have with each other, an impaired gut can dysregulate the brain and a dysregulated brain can impair digestive function. Thus it begins to make sense that around 60% of psychiatric patients, including a majority of those with depression, also complain of digestive issues. [31]

A 2020 article in the *Annals of Medicine* reported:

> *What is clear is that when we are depressed, the gut microbiome is often missing beneficial flora. If we can add those elements back in, maybe we can re-energize that cycle … increasing evidence that the Gut Microbiome (GM) and microbial dysbiosis [bad gut microbes] contribute to some of the more prevalent mental health and neurocognitive disorders, such as depression, anxiety, obsessive-compulsive disorder, post-traumatic stress disorder, schizophrenia, bipolar disorder, and dementia as well as the behavioural and psychological symptoms of dementia through the microbiota-gut-brain axis.* [32]

One study found that 'gut microbes of depressed patients are consistently found to be dysregulated' [33] and another that *'The comorbidity of depression and gut disease can be as high as 75%.'* [34]

Physical health and mental health depend on a healthy gut microbiome. Our gut microbes depend on us feeding them well and protecting them from harm.

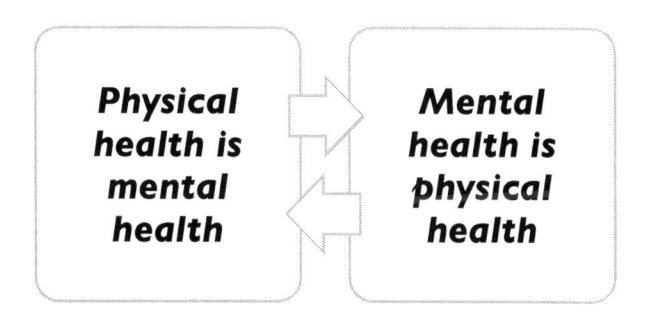

> **Physical health is mental health** ⇄ **Mental health is physical health**

An interesting example is how people who have had a bad bout of food poisoning are at much greater risk of a mental health disorder. Maybe that's not such a great revelation when you think how miserable it is to feel nauseous and utterly exhausted with projectile vomiting and explosive diarrhoea. But findings show that once people have passed this initial, acute phase and these major symptoms have cleared up completely, depression and anxiety still persist.

As I explore throughout this book, if something throws off our digestive system, and critically our healthy gut microbes, the whole body is more prone to poor regulation of nutrient and biochemical balance and chronic inflammation. These issues can happen in the body and in the brain, potentially resulting in poor mental health for years to come. Conditions such as irritable bowel syndrome (IBS), inflammatory bowel disease (IBD: colitis and Crohn's), chronic bloating, gastritis and gastroesophageal reflux disease (GERD) are inflammatory issues of the digestive tract that can impair our mental health too.

Our food choices affect how we function

Our abilities to concentrate, to process and retain new information, to master new skills and to manage our thoughts and feelings can all be affected by the foods we eat, when we eat, how we eat and what we don't eat, along with other lifestyle choices. Much of the chemical soup that regulates our brain function is manufactured or directly influenced by our digestive system. As the digestive system is, in turn, hugely influenced by what we eat and how well we process what we eat, then clearly every meal we consume could be either positively or negatively influencing both our gut health and our brain health. Time and again, mental health symptoms improve as the body gets healthier and deteriorate as we get ill. The connection between the two is becoming glaringly obvious:

> *For decades, researchers and doctors thought that anxiety and depression contributed to [digestive] problems. But our studies and others show that it may also be the other way around ... Researchers are finding evidence that irritation in the gastrointestinal system may send signals to the central nervous system that trigger mood changes ... These new findings may explain why a higher-than-normal percentage of people with IBS and functional bowel problems develop depression and anxiety.* [35]

Knowing this helps to make clear just how major a role our gut health plays in our mental well-being. It is hardly surprising that what we eat can change our experience of the world, because what we eat feeds our gut microbes and they are the master programmers of our mental health. And this is an exciting revelation: it means **we have agency over our mental health through making better decisions about what we eat and how we choose to live.**

In Part Two I delve into the gut microbiome's most favoured food sources: specific types of fibre found in some plant foods; polyphenols, also found in certain plants; and the fascinating alchemy of bug-rich fermented foods. Combine these functional, gut-healthy foods with the important practice of giving the gut a regular rest period with frequent fasting windows, and we are on track for better mental health. But first, a little more biology.

Short-chain fatty acids: Our gut bugs' thank-you gift

When we eat gut-friendly foods and reduce gut-toxic foods, our happy gut microbes reward us by producing compounds called short-chain fatty acids

(SCFAs), also known as postbiotics. These are super-fuel for the cells that line the gut, helping to keep our colon disease free and our intestinal lining healthy (not leaky). This is critical for good digestion, the maintenance of happy gut microbes and to prevent the immune system being inappropriately triggered – all very important stuff.

Recent findings have shown a more direct way in which SCFAs affect our mental status. If our gut microbes are well cared for, they produce sufficient SCFAs to heal not only the gut but the brain too. A certain type of SCFA called butyrate is now understood to be passed from the gut up to the brain, where it has anti-anxiety and anti-depressive effects while increasing levels of a brain chemical called BDNF (brain-derived neurotrophic factor, also known as fertiliser for the brain), which improves brain health and function. The sequence of events goes like this:

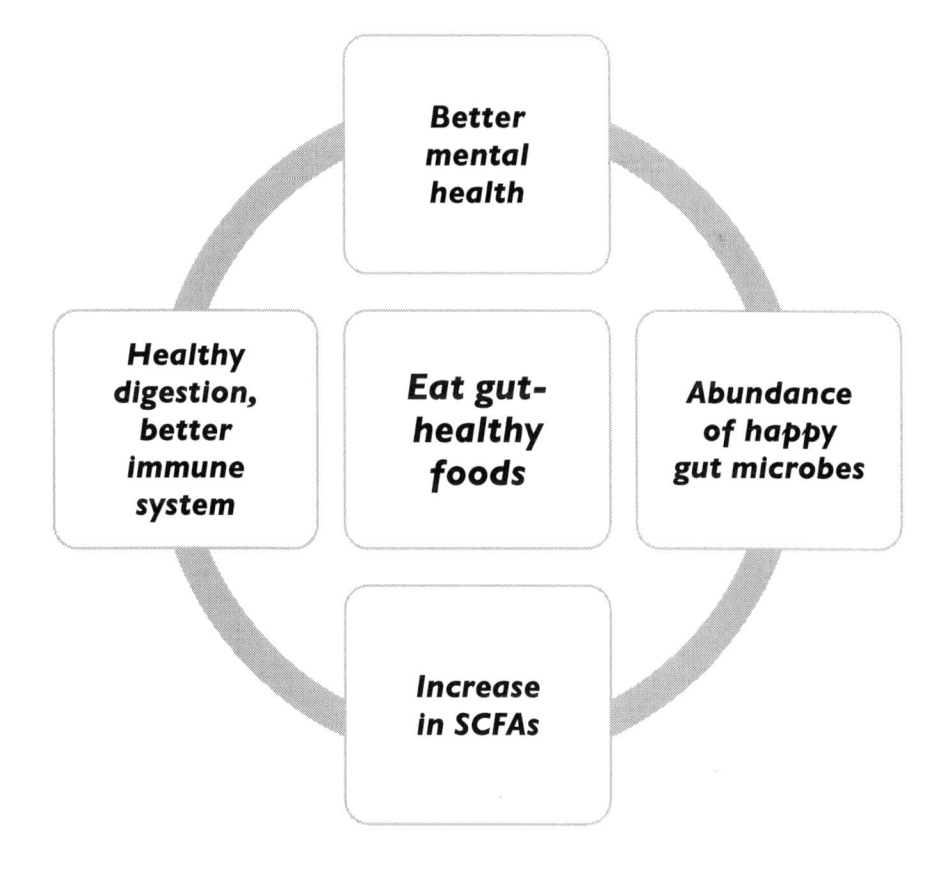

- **Eat gut-healthy foods**
- **Abundance of happy gut microbes**
- **Increase in SCFAs**
- **Healthy digestion, better immune system**
- **Better mental health**

There's lots more on SCFAs in Part Two, where you will learn how to support your own gut microbes to make more of these incredible, gut-healing, brain-balancing health bombs. But you might be wondering how on earth these gut-made gifts get up to the brain. That is why we need a quick look at the vagus nerve.

A short introduction to a very long nerve

The vagus nerve is a bi-directional communication superhighway where the gut bugs talk to the brain and the brain talks to the gut bugs. Depending on the state of our gut microbiome, that cross-talk can be fluent, supportive and calming, or disruptive, irritating and destabilising.

> **GEEK BOX**
>
> **The vagus nerve**
>
> *The vagus nerve is the 10th cranial nerve and the longest of them all. It gets its name from the Latin word vagus, meaning straying or wandering, because it 'wanders' around our organs. For people who have permanent damage to their vagus nerve or in some medical conditions such as epilepsy, a tiny pacemaker-like device can be inserted into the body to stimulate this nerve.*

The lanes of this superhighway aren't equally split between those going up and those coming down. The latest scientific studies show that in fact there are four times more lines of communication going up from the gut to the brain than there are coming down from the brain to the gut. That means four times more information is passing from the digestive tract up into our brain, directly influencing what our brain is doing, than is coming out of the brain, managing our digestive function.

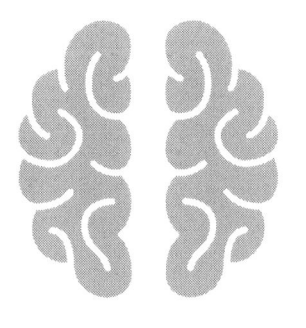

> **Four times more info is passed from the gut to the brain than from the brain to the gut**

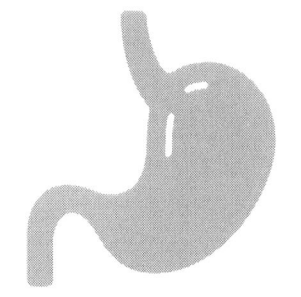

Our gut–brain communication is one of the main systems for managing brain inflammation, which as we've seen is the root cause of so much brain imbalance and mood disruption. It is enormously influential on how the different regions of the brain work in relation to the messages it sends out to the rest of the body, as well as how it communicates and regulates itself. This, of course, then influences how we feel, think and regulate our emotions and experiences.

Put another way, our gut health, influenced by our food and lifestyle choices, shapes the information coming out of our brain, which changes our perception of life, from our interpersonal relationships to our management of stress, to how well we get over illness and recover from trauma. Appetite, cravings, energy levels, mood regulation, stress resilience – all are largely to do with gut management. Ever wondered why we talk about a 'gut instinct' or 'having a feeling in my gut'? Our digestive health is such a major player in our entire life experience that it begs the question: Which is in control here, the gut or the brain? The science is not yet conclusive, but what is certain is that more recognition needs to be given to the enormous influence the gut microbiome has on all aspects of our health, well-being and sense of the world.

One major role of the vagus nerve is to send neurotransmitters (brain chemicals) or their precursor ingredients up to the brain from the gut, along with those happy, healing SCFAs made by our gut bugs. Remember, the brain depends on these chemicals coming from the gut to be able to function. Some neurotransmitters pass up ready formed, and others are made by the brain from the constituent parts that are made in the gut and passed up via the vagus nerve. GABA, our anti-anxiety, calm chemical; dopamine, which manages pleasure and motivation; acetylcholine, one of our most important neurotransmitters involved in mood, memory, sleep, motivation and stress management – all of these are made in the gut. Serotonin, our happy, confident chemical, is too; in fact, around 90% of the serotonin in our body is in our digestive tract, not our brain. Gut serotonin is an essential part of good digestion, helping to keep us regular and supporting happy gut microbes – further cementing the gut–brain connection to mental health.

Management of the vagus nerve is fundamental to good emotional and mental health and biological harmony. There are many reasons why this nerve may become faulty (called losing vagal tone), even if we eat well and work hard at nourishing our gut microbes. Loss of vagal tone causes a disruption in the brain's self-management and that of the digestive system, leading to constipation or diarrhoea, bloating, acid reflux, stomach cramps, disrupting appetite, energy levels and so much more. This can create an unhealthy environment in the digestive tract, causing the gut microbes to suffer, which then affects the messages going up to the brain via the vagus nerve. Now the brain's regulation systems are even more off and over time mental health suffers. This is why so many people with mental health issues have digestive issues and vice versa: the two systems are dependent on each other. Sustained poor vagal tone can also cause tight breathing, elevated heart rate and blood pressure, poor-quality sleep, slow recovery from exercise and illness, and ultimately an unhappy brain.

Loss of vagal tone

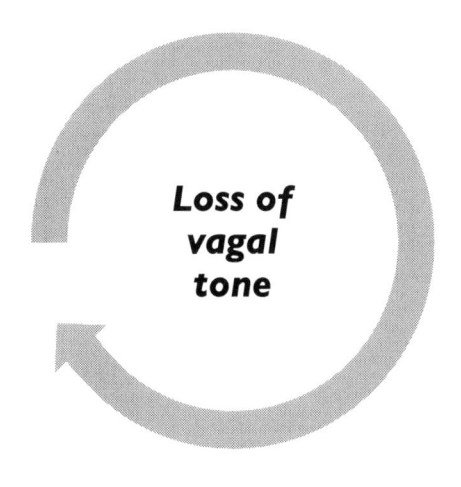

- Poor gut health
- Poor brain health
- Poor digestive health
- Poor nourishment to the brain
- Poor mental health

Chronic stress is a major culprit in poor vagal tone. Being overly stressed is an accepted part of modern life, yet it is so disruptive to our well-being, not least because stress overrides vagal nerve function, causing the gut–brain axis to be disrupted. Stress hormones are bullies. They have to be as they need to dominate when we are under threat as a priority over all other functions, when the stress hormones drive us to take action for self-preservation. Digestion, healing and immune function are turned off so we can fight off or flee from the enemy or freeze and pretend to be dead. Of course, as we saw in Chapter One, these are largely experiences from yesteryear, back in the days of living off the land and fending for ourselves. But this exact fight-or-flight stress system is now being triggered by a multitude of modern-day experiences that are no longer life threatening, but prompt the same high-alert crisis management response, to the detriment of our vagal tone.

Any unresolved trauma is perpetuating the fight-or-flight overresponse and suppressing our vagal tone.

Much of the communicating and regulating the vagus nerve is tasked with, from heart rate and blood pressure to stomach acid production, protein digestion, bowel function and everything in between, is dysregulated when we are in stress mode. Understanding this is critical if we are to get back in charge of our mental health balance. The stressors can be our thoughts, our food, the chemicals in our environment or a poorly gut and disrupted immune system – anything that causes the body's sensing systems to feel overwhelmed.

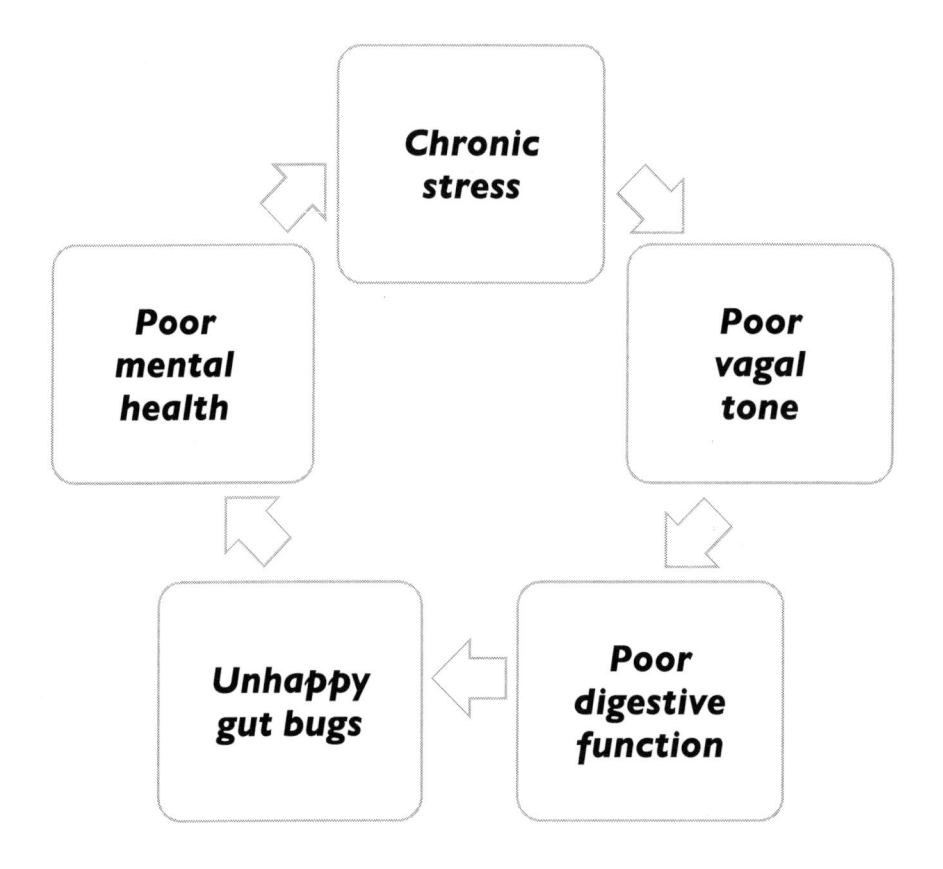

Chronic stress → **Poor vagal tone** → **Poor digestive function** → **Unhappy gut bugs** → **Poor mental health** → **Chronic stress**

Learning a few easy health hacks to help switch off the stress hormones when we feel tension and anxiety rising can start to reinstate a sense of control over our body and mind. Interrupting the incessant flow of stress hormones enables the vagus nerve to be activated, calming our nervous system and allowing our rest, recover and digest functions to be dominant. Then the brain can start to fine-tune, turning off crisis management responses, activating renewal of brain cells and calming inflammation. With that comes balance, harmony and a happier brain.

Becoming proficient in these techniques is a key strategy in your happy brain pursuits, so you'll find some vagal tone exercises in Chapter Nine.

A poignant case history

Let me illustrate the kind of changes you can hope to achieve with an example. Several years ago I worked with a young man who came to stay for three weeks on a residential gut health programme I was running. His concerned parents were paying for him in the hope he would lose some weight and get some energy back, which would then allow him to feel better about himself. Let's call him Peter. Very overweight and subdued, Peter didn't engage that much. He was quiet, private and appeared rather bewildered at being there.

Over the weeks we met and talked numerous times. Initially we looked at his diet and lifestyle – several cans of soda daily, lots of takeaways, burgers and fries in particular. He used to be sporty but now barely even walked anywhere. We then began to talk about his life, his aspirations, what gave him joy. Peter couldn't find much to look forward to and felt doomed to life always being a struggle. He didn't know why, he just felt he wasn't good enough. He talked about his body being his prison and his mind being his jailor. He had been on antidepressants but had chosen to stop as he couldn't tolerate the side effects. He felt nothing very much, mostly despair and misery. He was clearly very depressed.

The programme Peter was on was a group stay where participants had daily health talks; the food was wholesome, tasty, full of good fats, fibre, live foods and protein, with an acute focus on optimising digestion and the gut microbiome in particular. Thanks to the great chefs, the food was enjoyable, not punitive. There were also two days a week of no breakfast, a big hearty lunch and a mug of bone broth in the evening – a gentle style of fasting.

Peter struggled at first. He craved sugar, his diet drinks and the comfort of his constant snacking. He had even less energy. He didn't plan to stay. Thankfully he did, with lots of support from the health and medical team. We kept a close eye on him and reminded him what was going on – his body was having to reroute from having a constant supply of sugar to managing without all that fast and inflammatory fuel and turn to slow, steady fat burning instead.

Being young and male helped Peter. His body was able to adapt relatively quickly. By the time he left three weeks later, he had lost 8 kg; a real success. However, there was a far more significant shift for him. He felt better about himself because he had lost weight, but what really allowed him to leave us with true positivity, a spring in his step and a smile on his face was hope. I will never forget his parting thank-you to the team: 'For the first time in my life I am waking up feeling hopeful.'

Peter's brain was beginning to course-correct thanks to a major dietary clean-up, removing the daily inflammatory foods and drinks and eating meals that nourished his body and brain while allowing his blood sugar to normalise and his gut microbes to thrive. That's why he lost so much weight and that's also why he left with a much happier brain.

Take a deep breath and get ready for your very own happy brain action plan in Part Two.

PART TWO
THE HAPPY BRAIN ACTION PLAN

Here we go... Keep this in mind:

The act of choosing to eat nourishing foods is, in itself, healing.

I'll start with a warning: don't try and do too much too quickly. There are a lot of small changes you can implement one by one that will get you on the path to a happier brain. It's important to see this as a process, a practice even, something you work on gradually and continue to experiment with for your lifetime. What every individual needs will be slightly different – one change might be a major needle-shifter within days or weeks for some, while for others it has no tangible effect. So, take things slowly, be curious, be patient and understand that even if you don't notice an improvement, something good is still happening within you, one nudge at a time. Fixing the body takes longer than merely suppressing symptoms with medication.

The compounding or cumulative result of small changes over time – known as the butterfly effect – is fundamental to long-term resolution of health issues, including mental health. Very few people can make several radical changes all at once and stick to them. Don't add to your current mental health challenges by setting yourself up for failure. Instead, pick one or two of the recommendations here that you consider most doable, find a way to integrate them into your daily habits and, once it no longer feels like an effort, once the change or changes fit comfortably into your daily routine, then look for another small change you can start to implement.

If you're reading this feeling a little cynical, maybe thinking that what you eat can't possibly have any significant impact on your anxiety or depression, think again. The Royal Australian and New Zealand College of Psychiatry now states in its clinical guidelines that it is *'non-negotiable'* that lifestyle medicine – *'adopting healthy sleep habits ... [and] the institution of a healthy diet and regular exercise'* – is the foundation for the effective management of mood disorders. [36]

Our body is a highly integrated and complex set of systems. All of these systems need food and more specifically nutrients to function well. It is universally accepted that a healthy diet (many studies reference the Mediterranean diet as the gold standard) can reduce the risk of cardiovascular disease, diabetes, cancer, auto-immune disease and chronic digestive disorders, so why is it so much harder to accept that the brain might benefit too?

CHAPTER FIVE
Your Gut Health *Is* Your Brain Health

Step 1. The big first step: Cut the junk

It's probably not news to you that highly processed 'junk' food not only contains little to no nourishment, it is actually damaging to the gut microbes and many other systems in the body, including the happy balance of the brain. Packaged foods that have gone through multiple food processing systems, have long shelf lives and multiple unpronounceable ingredients should be an occasional, rare feature of your diet. This really is non-negotiable. However, it can be a challenge when these foods provide instant, albeit fleeting pleasure and are so ubiquitous. Remind yourself of the deep connection between what we eat and how we feel, think and function to help you stay away from those foods that might be disrupting your delicate gut and brain balance.

The simple starting message for your happy brain action plan is to **eat (and drink) more fresh, whole foods and fewer packaged, highly processed foods.** The latter include most snack and convenience foods such as many breakfast cereals, potato and corn-based snacks such as crisps and tortilla chips, sweets, ready-made sauces, ready meals especially those with crispy/breaded coatings, deep-fried foods and anything artificially flavoured. Beverage choices are important too: fizzy drinks, energy drinks, squashes and alcohol are all problematic if consumed to excess. I give some easy swaps later in the chapter.

I'm not saying all these foods are awful, but most are and none is good for you. If you do currently eat them, eat fewer of them less often and combine them with more wholesome foods. Take a look at the ingredient list: if there are more than five ingredients and/or ingredients you can't pronounce or wouldn't find in your kitchen, it's probably a no.

Be honest with yourself. There are many occasions when we eat 'grab and go' foods, which tend to be more 'junkie', without even clocking it, such as grabbing a packet of something when paying for fuel; automatically taking a couple of biscuits with your mid-afternoon cuppa; or mindlessly eating sweets or snacks when watching TV.

Refined carbs aka fast carbs and high-starch foods

I sum these up as the GPS: Grains, Potatoes and Sweet-tasting foods. This doesn't mean you can never have rice, bread, potatoes or something sweet, it's about being aware that these foods may be having a negative impact on your metabolic and mental regulation. Cutting these foods out or down, at least for a while, will allow you to find out if you feel better without them. You can then make an informed choice about what to eat more of and what to avoid.

Some of the main culprits are often a feature of highly processed foods. A great place to start is to greatly reduce your consumption of sugar and refined grains. Broadly speaking that's things made with flour and/or sugar, like biscuits, cakes, white bread, pastries, breakfast cereals, flavoured yogurts, milk and white chocolate (dark chocolate has some health benefits), snack/'health' bars and most sodas and squashes. These foods and drinks are very aggressive on blood glucose levels and, as we saw in Chapter Two, blood sugar peaks and troughs can be really problematic for a happy brain.

Again, take it slowly, especially if you ordinarily eat a lot of sweet foods and refined grains. Give your body time to adapt otherwise you could feel even worse, making it so much harder to continue.

As your blood sugar begins to normalise and your taste buds adjust, you may find you naturally start to eat a wider range of happy brain foods to fill the gaps the sugary foods and refined grains have been occupying in your diet. You will probably miss the momentary pleasure and burst of energy your favourite sweet and processed foods were providing, but most people are amazed at how quickly they notice the physical and mental benefits, which make continuing to stay off them so much easier.

Online resources for lower-carb recipes and healthier food swaps are abundant. Search for an ingredient or dish you love and simply preface it with 'low-carb'. You'll be amazed at all the ingenious low-grain, non-grain, low-starch and low-sugar alternatives there are.

Easy swaps for increasing your healthier carbs
- Bean or lentil pasta in place of wheat pasta
- Sourdough bread rather than sliced white bread
- Sourdough rye bread in place of wheat bread
- Sweet potato in place of white potato (sweet potatoes are more nutritious and more slowly digested due to their higher fibre content)
- Sweet potato wraps rather than wheat wraps
- Roasted nuts in place of potato crisps and corn chips
- Chickpea crackers rather than wheat-based crackers
- Slices of aubergine and/or courgette in place of lasagne sheets
- Cauliflower rice rather than normal rice
- Portobello mushrooms in place of burger buns
- Natural yogurt with fresh fruit rather than sweetened fruit yogurt
- Natural yogurt, berries, nuts and seeds in place of breakfast cereals
- Sparkling or soda water with a squeeze of lime or lemon rather than cordials or sweet sodas
- Low-sugar kombucha for a gut-healthy fizzy drink in place of sodas or alcohol

The nutritional ketogenic diet

Much of the current research in metabolic psychiatry refers to a ketogenic diet as an intervention for mental health conditions. A ketogenic diet is high in fat (approximately 60% of calories), moderate in protein (30%) and very low in carbohydrates (10%),[37] generally regarded as 50 g of carbohydrates or lower per day. This is roughly equivalent to just two slices of bread, a small bowl of pasta or rice, three medium-sized potatoes, two medium apples or roughly 1½ bananas as a total daily intake of carbohydrates.

As you can see, it takes very little to exceed the daily carbohydrate limit and this can therefore be difficult to adhere to successfully. The reason for such a low carb count is to force the body into a state of ketosis, where it is keeping blood glucose low enough to be constantly producing ketones from burning body fat and/or fats from food. This is the protocol that has been used for over 100 years for people with treatment-resistant seizure disorders. As discussed in Chapter Two, the brain runs very well on ketones as its main fuel source and doing so appears to be profoundly beneficial to those people whose have exclusively fat-loving brains.

The good news is that significant improvements are seen in those who simply reduce their carbohydrate levels without going to the extremes of a fully ketogenic diet. The recommendations I give in this book focus on a lowish-carbohydrate way of eating. Our bodies are designed to be dual-fuel burners, running off glucose after a meal and turning to body fat to make ketones between meals and at night. When we can do this well, we are metabolically flexible. That is a healthy state to achieve and once we are there the body is making ketones, just not on a constant basis as it does on a full ketogenic diet. Some people may need to be in full ketosis before they experience significant benefit to their mental health, but most do not. If you are interested in trying a fully ketogenic diet rather than the less extreme low-carbohydrate recommendations I provide, do seek professional advice to ensure you are doing it correctly and safely.

> *N.B.: Nutritional ketosis is very different to diabetic ketoacidosis, a dangerous condition experienced in poorly managed type 1 diabetes.*

Step 2. Getting going on your gut health

All of the top five leading causes of death (heart disease followed by cancer, lung and brain diseases) in the Western world are lifestyle driven and they all have one underlying common trigger: chronic inflammation. As I explained in Chapter Three, what we eat has a huge influence over our levels of systemic inflammation, including in the brain. This is why diet is as helpful to an unhappy brain as it is to an ailing body.

One of the main inflammatory management systems in the body is the gut microbiome, those billions of microbes that live in our intestine (look back to Chapter Four for more). These microbes are profoundly affected by what we choose to eat, or not eat. Meal by meal we can be helping or harming our gut microbes.

A happy gut means a happy brain, and a happy gut needs to be fed well.

Nurture your gut microbes using the 3Fs

So what does nurturing your gut microbes look like? Remove (reduce) the substances that kill off your good gut bugs – step 1 – and feed your gut microbes what your they require to thrive – step 2. It's really not that complicated.

And what your gut microbes need to work well can be summed up in the 3Fs:

- Fibre and polyphenols
- Fermented foods
- Fasting

In step 1 you removed some of the more gut-harmful products such as processed and sugary foods. In this step you can begin to focus on the 3Fs. If all three are too much for you at the moment, start with just one – any one, they all work together – and that will begin your shift towards a happier gut and brain.

F1: Fibre and polyphenols

Your gut microbes' favourite fuel is fibre and polyphenols, substances found in many different plant foods. The main fibre-rich food groups are fruits and vegetables, nuts and seeds, beans, lentils and mushrooms (I'll explain what polyphenols are later).

Human beings can't digest fibre, meaning it can't pass into the body via the intestinal wall, it stays in the digestive system largely unchanged. However, not only can our gut bugs digest fibre, they rely on it. Fibre is what fuels our gut microbes and allows them to do all the wondrous things they do for the benefit of our physical and mental health. This is why fibre is termed prebiotic: it is the fuel for probiotics, another term for our healthy gut microbes.

Consuming more fibre in general has been associated with benefits for many chronic diseases from obesity to type 2 diabetes, some cancers and digestive issues. The NHS, the British Heart Foundation, the British Nutrition Foundation and Heart UK all support the idea of increasing fibre in the diet. The consensus amount among health experts is at least 30 g of fibre per day for adults – we'll look at what that means in practice in a moment. Most adults are getting around half that recommended amount. In 2005 fibre was classed as 'a nutrient of concern' by the Dietary Guidelines for Americans after studies found that nine out of ten adults were considerably under-consuming fibre. And even meeting the 30 g target gets us nowhere close to the fibre content we were likely consuming with a hunter-gatherer lifestyle, which is estimated to have been around 150 g a day.

How much fibre do you need?

So a sensible amount to aim for is 30 g of fibre a day. You want to be getting this from as wide a variety of foods as possible to ensure lots of different types to feed your own individual gut microbial families. If you are prone to bloating and/or irritable bowel issues, increase your fibre intake slowly to give your gut microbes time to adjust.

What does 30 g of fibre look like? Here's a quick guide to good sources of fibre – we'll look at the different types later in the chapter:

- 2 tablespoons of soaked chia seeds = 10 g
- 2 tablespoons of soaked ground flaxseeds = 4 g
- 4 tablespoons of cooked lentils = 8 g
- ½ avocado = 5 g
- 5 broccoli florets = 4 g
- 4 tablespoons of cooked spinach = 4 g
- 4 tablespoons of cooked peas = 7 g
- ½ can of chickpeas or butter beans = 15 g
- 4 tablespoons of cooked oats = 4 g
- 1 medium banana = 3 g
- 1 small apple = 3 g
- 4 heaped tablespoons or 125 g of cooked quinoa = 3 g
- 1 medium carrot = 3 g
- 3 tablespoons of cooked brown rice = 2 g

As you can see, it takes quite a lot of food to get to 30 g per day. It's also a tedious process to count up these fibre grams. Instead, use the simple principle of adding a range of high-fibre foods to every meal you eat, paying particular attention to foods that have high fibre by weight and lots of natural colour. These foods are:

- Beans and lentils
- Whole fruits and vegetables, especially if you include the skin on fresh produce such as sweet potato, butternut squash, apple or kiwi fruit
- Soaked high-fibre seeds like chia, flax and psyllium husk

Rather than sticking to the standard recommendation of five servings of fruit and vegetables a day, think instead about seven, divided 5:2 – 5 servings of vegetables and 2 servings of fruit per day. A simple gauge for a standard serving of vegetables is roughly the size of your fist – larger if the food is light and leafy like lettuce and smaller if it's very dense like lentils.

Another useful visual method is to fill at least half your plate or bowl with high-fibre foods:

- A big mixed salad and some steamed broccoli to accompany a stew, chilli or omelette
- A range of roasted veggies such as red onions, courgette, aubergine, peppers, skin-on sweet potatoes – throw in a few handfuls of spinach with a tin of lentils or beans to make a super-charged high-fibre, nutrient-dense dish to have alongside some meat, fish, eggs or tofu
- 2 tablespoons of chia and flax seeds soaked overnight to make a loose gloop, mixed with berries or chopped kiwi fruit, live yogurt and coconut flakes for a high-fibre breakfast bowl

A note on fruit

We don't need fruit to be healthy, so if you're not a fan, don't worry. All the nutrients we get from fruit can be found in vegetables. If you do enjoy fruit, here are some simple principles to make sure you're not overdoing the natural sugars. Modern fruit is grown to be very sweet, so too much can be a problem.

- Always stick to whole fruits as opposed to juiced fruits (unless you have a health reason requiring juicing). As soon as you start peeling, juicing or blending fruit (berries are an exception), you are removing or altering the fibre and other compounds your gut microbes require to thrive. Much of what is good for us in plant foods, and fruit in particular, comes from the plant's self-protection system against insects and microbes, which is on and just under the skin. If you peel a fruit, you lose a lot of that natural power. However, if a fruit has been heavily sprayed with pesticides while it grows, the spray deters the attackers, so the plant doesn't have to make its own deterrent. Therefore, for any fruit that can be eaten skin on – apples, pears, berries, stone fruits, even kiwi – aim wherever possible to buy organic and simply wash and eat whole. A little vinegar in water is a great fruit and veg wash.
- Aim for two pieces (or two handfuls) of lower-sugar fruits (apples, pears, plums, kiwi fruit, berries, citrus fruits).
- Ripe tropical fruit like mangos, pineapple and bananas are high in sugar and easy to overeat. Underripe tropical fruit such as green mangos, greenish bananas or firm papayas are not nearly so sweet and contain some gut-healthy fibre, so can be added to salads and yogurt dishes.
- It's best to have your fruit servings earlier in the day and serve with other food or after a meal to ensure the fruit sugars are less disruptive.

Types of fibre

Not all fibre is the same. There are two main categories: insoluble fibre (aka roughage) and soluble fibre, which dissolves in water. Most natural, whole plant foods contain some insoluble and some soluble fibre. These terms are gradually being phased out as the understanding of the structures and functions of different types of fibre deepens. Currently over 100 different types of fibre have been identified, with sub-categories referring to whether the fibre is fermented by bacteria; is used to bulk the stool; has the capacity to slow the release of sugars into the blood; reduces absorption of cholesterol into the blood; or has a laxative effect.

Insoluble fibre is largely made up of indigestible cellulose, the main substance constituting the cell walls of plants giving them their structure, like our skeleton – it's tough. Insoluble fibre can be helpful to keep transit time (the time it takes for your food to pass through you) at an optimal rate: too fast and you don't have time to absorb enough nutrients from your food and you are likely to have loose stools; too slow and the bad gut bugs can build up, causing bloating and constipation, while toxins that should be expelled can be reabsorbed. Transit time can range from a few hours to several days, even for the same person. Recent research suggests that optimal transit time is less than 24 hours and those who achieve this tend to have better gut microbial diversity.

Transit Time and Bowel Function

Transit time is the time it takes from food being eaten to its being passed out in the stool. Anywhere from 12 to 48 hours is generally considered 'normal'. Food passes through the digestive tract at different rates depending on where it is in the system. The stomach holds food for 2–5 hours. This is where the contents are churned up with stomach acid and enzymes to break down proteins. The more protein there is in a meal, the longer it is held in the stomach. Transit through the small intestine can be anywhere from 2 to 6 hours, where the partially digested food is further digested and then nutrients are released from the intestine into the bloodstream. It can take anywhere from 10 to 59 [38] hours for the remaining food to pass through the large intestine, home to most of our gut microbes. This is where the fermentation of fibre and production of postbiotics happens.

Structural differences, food choices and hydration levels, digestive signalling via the vagus nerve and stress levels can all affect an individual's transit time. Both too long and too short a time can be an issue. How can you find out your transit time? Note the time of day, swallow some whole kernels of sweetcorn without chewing them (not advised on a regular basis) and look out for the kernels coming out the other end. A good serving of beetroot is another way to check your transit time, as it will turn your poop purple-red.

Why is this important? Healthy bowel movements, generally agreed to be an easy and complete evacuation of bowels at least once daily without urgency or straining, is indicative of a healthy environment within the digestive tract, conducive to a healthy microbiome and all the wider health benefits associated with healthy gut bugs. An overgrowth of unhealthy gut bugs can cause constipation and constipation can cause an unhealthy overgrowth of gut microbes. Chronic (ongoing) constipation is associated with systemic inflammation and many other health issues as it represents imbalance and dysfunction within the gut. If you are not having regular bowel movements daily, you will be retaining matter – dead microbes, undigested fibre, toxins, pathogens, even hormones that the body wants to eliminate. If you aren't moving this matter out, you could be reabsorbing things that should be expelled. Human faecal matter is largely water, hence if you are dehydrated you may not be having good and regular bowel movements. Similarly, if you have a low fibre diet your gut microbes may not be functioning well, creating issues with bowel movements.

Watery, loose stools that are frequent and urgent also indicate an unhappy gut. This can be caused by poor food quality, foods that aren't being *digested well, inflammation within the intestine and an overgrowth of unhelpful gut bugs. If you are living with slow and sluggish or unformed, runny poops, this is a strong sign that you need to work on your gut health, which in turn could have a transformative effect on many other aspects of your physical and mental health. Remember, a happy brain is a happy gut.*

We can benefit from a little insoluble fibre regularly to keep things moving, but too much can be irritating to the gut (I liken it to wire wool going through your system). This is especially true for those who have existing gut issues, as in irritable bowel syndrome (IBS), which around 20% of the UK population suffer with and is often correlated to mental health disorders. Insoluble fibre is not used as a fuel for our gut bugs, so there's no need to be forcing down bowlfuls of bran – a little goes a long way. You'll get plenty from eating whole fruit, vegetables, nuts and seeds.

GEEK BOX

What's in all that poop?

Your poop not only includes waste food products and indigestible fibre. Anywhere up to 60% is old, dead gut bacteria – roughly 100 billion per gram of stool. The turnover of our gut bugs is vast, hence we need to be looking after them every day.

Soluble fibre is the type of fibre you really want to focus on. Most whole foods naturally contain this type of fibre. After eating it dissolves in water, becoming a slimy, soothing goo full of mucilage, great for gut wall healing, a healthy transit time and gut microbe feeding. Soluble fibre-rich foods help us feel full, help regulate blood sugar levels, can play a role in balancing blood fats and, of course, fuel our busy gut bugs.

Foods high in particularly beneficial types of soluble fibre include:

- The allium family of vegetables: red and white onions, shallots, spring onions, leeks, chives and garlic. Even small amounts can be helpful. Raw or cooked, they have anti-inflammatory, antioxidant and immune-supporting properties too, so they deserve superfood status
- Brassicas: broccoli, cauliflower, all the different cabbages, kale, bok choy and turnips. Cooking these veggies makes them easier to digest and more nutritious than eating them raw
- Pulses: beans, especially black beans, and all types of lentils
- Flax and chia seeds if pre-soaked
- Avocados
- Sweet potatoes
- Apples, pears and kiwi fruit

Prebiotic fibre

One type of soluble fibre stands out as a real gut-healthy hero: prebiotic fibre – fibre that specifically feeds our beneficial gut microbes. Various sources have been identified and studied, some of which are naturally found in common foods and others that can be used in supplement form as they don't readily feature in useful quantities in our diet.

Foods particularly high in prebiotic fibre are:

- Leeks, onions and garlic
- Asparagus
- Mushrooms
- Chicory root (or any bitter leaf) and the root of romaine lettuce
- Most pulses: beans and lentils
- Jerusalem artichokes

- Globe artichokes
- Savoy cabbage

GEEK BOX

Activating your garlic

There is an immune-boosting super-compound called allicin that you can get from eating garlic, but you need to activate its production. Finely chop, grate or crush your garlic and leave it to sit for around 15 minutes before cooking with it. As the oxygen in the air hits the broken-up garlic cells, an enzymic reaction occurs that creates lots of allicin.

This type of fibre can be challenging for some people as it can create excess bloating and wind. This doesn't mean it isn't beneficial for you, but it most likely means you don't have the correct types or a large enough number of the microbes that ferment the specific kind of prebiotic fibre that causes you trouble. Most commonly the problem foods are garlic and onions, beans and lentils. If you know that some of these are causing you to bloat excessively, avoid them for a while and focus on building up your tolerance with the other 2Fs, ideally for 8–12 weeks. Then try small amounts of the troublesome foods and see how you get on. Hopefully you will then have increased your range of gut bugs. Start with small amounts, chew really well and employ some of the other digestion-supporting tips I discuss later, and you should find you can gradually tolerate more and more as your beneficial, prebiotic fibre–loving bacterial species grow more numerous.

GEEK BOX

Prebiotic fibre for sleep

Prebiotic fibre, specifically inulin and green banana powder, has been shown to help increase the amount of deep sleep for those with sleep issues.

Resistant starch

Another favourite fuel source for our gut microbes is resistant starch. This is a form of starchy carbohydrate that resists digestion, reaching our large intestine undigested. There it is used as a particularly potent prebiotic for our probiotics to feed on.

Most pulses contain good levels of resistant starch. However, if you struggle with digesting beans and lentils, an easy way to increase your resistant starch intake is to cook and cool certain high-starch foods such as potatoes, oats, pasta and quinoa (a pseudo-grain, actually a seed but looks and behaves like a grain). If they are freshly cooked and eaten straight away, these starchy foods are readily digested and absorbed as glucose, which can spike blood sugar, hence I suggest people reduce or avoid potatoes and grains as a general rule. But if these foods are cooked, cooled for at least six hours and then eaten cold or reheated, they go through a rather magical process where the starches fold in a different way, known as starch retrogradation. Starch retrogradation causes much of this starch to change into resistant starch – that is, resistant to our digestion – so it stays in the gut, travelling down to the large intestine and fuelling our gut microbes, which makes it not only great for our gut, it also has a much lower impact on blood sugar levels.

Foods high in resistant starch are:

- Very pale yellow, still slightly green bananas
- Cooked and cooled starchy vegetables such as potatoes, sweet potatoes and parsnips
- Cooked and cooled whole oats
- Cooked and cooled rice (be careful to reheat really well to avoid food poisoning)
- Beans and lentils
- Potato starch powder, which can be used in cooking or added to yogurt or smoothies to increase your resistant starch levels easily

Polyphenols

Polyphenols aren't strictly speaking fibre but are found in many fibre-rich plant foods. Over 8,000 of these protective plant compounds have so far been identified. They are used by growing plants as natural sunscreens and pesticides – when we eat the plant, we get the benefits. As well as exerting anti-inflammatory and cell-protecting effects, certain polyphenols have been shown to be favourite foods for our beneficial gut microbes. Although they're still not fully understood, it's thought these compounds help keep bad gut bugs at bay while encouraging the growth of some of the good guys.

In particular, polyphenols fuel up some of the keystone gut microbes, meaning the most abundant and supportive types of microbes that encourage the growth of many of the other microbial strains. These important keystone species thrive on a daily dose (or several) of polyphenol-rich foods. Some specific polyphenol families you may recognise are flavonoids (apples, berries, cherries and citrus fruits), catechins (green tea), resveratrol (red grape skins, red wine), isoflavones (soy) and lignans (flax seeds). Polyphenol-rich foods tend to be bitter tasting, like green tea, coffee, raw cacao, peppery olive oil and chicory root, or richly coloured, like berries, oranges, red peppers and turmeric.

Some of the richest food sources of polyphenols are:

- Spices: turmeric, ginger, clove, cinnamon
- Herbs: rosemary, parsley, coriander, basil, thyme, oregano
- Raw cacao and unsweetened cocoa
- Berries, especially blueberries, blackcurrants, redcurrants and raspberries
- Pomegranates
- Good-quality coffee and tea, especially matcha green tea
- Flax seeds (ground and soaked)
- Peppery olive oil
- Black seed oil (from black cumin seeds)

- Pistachios, pecans, hazelnuts and almonds
- Black beans and lentils
- Rye flour
- Broccoli and cauliflower
- Orange and red vegetables like sweet potatoes, butternut squash, carrots, orange peppers, beetroot, radishes, tomatoes, red onions

Again, there's no need to overthink this. If you go for a variety of colours and a wide range of fruits and veggies, nuts and seeds, beans and lentils, along with a liberal array of herbs and spices and good-quality olive oil, you will be getting different fibres, resistant starch and polyphenols as well as vitamins, minerals and tons of flavour. With an abundance of these foods you will ensure you keep your mental health-supporting gut microbes happy.

F2: Fermented foods

Fermented foods are nothing new. There is evidence of alcoholic beverages, made from the fermentation of rice and honey, as far back at 7000 BC. Historically fermentation was used to avoid food waste in the eras before refrigeration. It was essential to turn a glut of summer cabbages into a winter's worth of sauerkraut through the simple method of salting and soaking the shredded cabbage. An excess of milk, which would spoil within days or even hours pre-refrigeration, can last weeks and months as kefir, yogurt or cheese. This was an economic necessity before modern methods of food preservation such as canning, chemical preservation, freezing and pasteurisation. Countries around the world have their own traditional fermented dishes, which in many cases continue to be eaten daily even though the practical need to preserve foods no longer exists.

Many common foods and drinks have gone through a process of fermentation. Tea, coffee, chocolate and bread require fermentation, but these foods don't retain the living microbes that are produced over the long term. Fermentation in the context I'm discussing here refers to living foods and drinks, where the microbes that created them are still alive when you come to consume them. Depending on what is being fermented and whether a starter culture is added or wild fermentation is taking place, fermentation creates different beneficial microbes. Whichever way it happens, millions of beneficial microbes, mostly bacteria and yeasts, can be present in a single serving of fermented food or drink and they play an important role in allowing the gut microbiome to thrive.

Studies show that consuming fermented foods can increase the diversity of gut microbes and help regulate the immune system. Some fermented foods reduce inflammation and some appear to stimulate growth of the gut microbes already living in the gut as they pass through. Despite increasingly sophisticated testing, knowing precisely what is happening in an individual's gut microbiome is still an impossible quest. However, if after a few months of consuming fermented foods your physical and/or mental health symptoms are improving, that's a pretty good sign that the fermented foods are doing you some good.

Types of ferments

Traditional fermented foods around the world include sauerkraut (fermented cabbage) in Germany, Austria and Eastern Europe; kimchi (fermented spicy vegetables) in Korea; hàkarl (fermented shark meat) in Iceland; and soy sauce, miso and tempeh among many fermented soy products in Japan. Many countries have fermented forms of dairy, including a vast array of cheeses and different forms of live yogurt and soured, thickened milk products. Dairy kefir, a highly fermented milk drink, is one of the most microbially diverse and therefore beneficial forms of ferments, now widely available commercially and very easy to make at home. Dairy kefir is like yogurt on steroids (in a good way!), more sour and runnier with a slight fizz. It has different and more numerous strains of microbes than live natural yogurt and in far higher numbers. It has even been shown to help those who have issues digesting dairy become more tolerant to dairy. [39]

If you are travelling in foreign countries or even different regions of your own country, see if you can source some traditional fermented foods to help introduce new tastes and new gut bugs into your system. You can also have a go at making your own ferments. Many are extremely quick and simple to make, although it takes time for the magic process of fermentation to occur, from days to weeks depending on what you are fermenting. A good yogurt can be made in around 12 hours; dairy kefir takes more like 24–36 hours; sauerkraut and other fermented veggie mixes take around 2–3 weeks; while mature cheeses can take many months, even years.

It is worth noting that the fermented products such as sauerkraut that are available in some supermarkets and specialist shops may have been pasteurised (heat treated). This allows the product to be shelf-stable, meaning it can be stored without refrigeration for a long time without spoiling. However, the pasteurisation kills off all the live bacteria, good and bad, so a pasteurised sauerkraut or kimchi will not have any live beneficial microbes. Look for products that say 'raw' or 'unpasteurised' on the label, which will be in the chiller cabinets only. The pasteurised products may still have some benefit thanks to zombie microbes (see the Geek Box), but it's impossible to know for sure.

GEEK BOX

Zombie probiotics

These may sound scary, but in fact they're pretty cool. Heat-killed beneficial bacteria, officially called paraprobiotics, are beneficial microbes found in fermented foods that have been killed by heat, such as the live microbes that make the culture used to ferment the dough for sourdough bread. Although the mechanism isn't yet clear, it appears that despite no longer being active, these dead microbes may continue to offer some benefit. Some studies are finding a positive impact on the innate immune system and they appear to help keep pathogenic, nasty gut bugs at bay while having antioxidant and anti-inflammatory effects. [40]

Apple cider vinegar (ACV) is one of my favourite fermented foods. It needs to be raw and unpasteurised (often labelled as containing 'the mother', meaning the mother culture). It's an easy, great addition to dressings and is a digestive tonic. Never consume it neat, rather add between 1 teaspoon and 1 tablespoon to a small glass of water and knock it back just before you begin your meal.

Kombucha is a fermented tea drink where sweetened tea is added to a special culture, which consumes and ferments the added sugar. The culture (a SCOBY – symbiotic combination of bacteria and yeast) uses the sugar as fuel and in so doing ferments the tea, producing a drink filled with beneficial microbes. With a slight fizz and sour, tangy taste, it's served cold and is a great alternative to sodas and sports drinks. It's a lot more interesting than plain water while also doing you good.

These drinks have become readily available and some will be better quality than others. If you try a kombucha and it tastes very sweet, it hasn't been fermented for long enough or the SCOBY wasn't active enough. It's not the sugar you want, it's the result of the SCOBY eating up the sugar and turning the tea sour and microbially rich. You can try leaving an overly sweet kombucha for a day or two at room temperature to permit more fermentation to take place, reducing the remaining sugar. Do release the cap so gas can escape, as fermenting produces carbon dioxide and if it can't get out the bottle could explode.

Gut-friendly fermented foods

The most gut-friendly fermented foods are:

- Dairy: natural, sugar-free, live yogurt, dairy kefir, raw milk and/or mature cheeses, labneh (cheese made from strained yogurt)
- Raw vegetables: sauerkraut, kimchi, brined olives
- Drinks: water kefir, coconut kefir, kombucha

- Condiments: unfiltered raw apple cider vinegar, miso, umeboshi (Japanese pickled plums)
- Others: coconut or other 'mylk' yogurt, tempeh, fermented tofu, natto (fermented soy beans), traditionally made charcuterie

As with prebiotics, despite the immense positives associated with long-term use of these functional foods, some people experience pain and bloating after eating them, especially if eaten in large quantities in the early stages of introducing them. This is a sign that your gut microbes are not well balanced, so if you react badly, introduce small amounts, one at a time, gradually increase the amount and if symptoms persist, get some professional advice.

F3: Fasting

The third F to try to incorporate in your happy brain action plan is some fasting, or more precisely intermittent fasting, also called time-restricted eating. This simply entails consuming no calories from food or drink for 12 hours or longer. It's a highly effective and simple strategy for giving your digestive system a chance to rest and recover from the toll of daily digestion and for your gut microbes to regulate and proliferate. While food, even the healthiest of foods, is passing through your small and large intestines, a degree of wear and tear will be taking place.

As with everything I'm recommending, start slowly. Most people naturally fast throughout the night. However, now that food has become so much easier to access throughout the day and night, there has been a trend for the average non-eating – aka fasting – window to get shorter. Rather than finishing the evening meal by 6–7 pm and then consuming no calories (food or drink) until 6–7 am the next day, which creates a natural fasting window of around 12 hours, many people today rarely make it to 8–10 hours.

It is really important to keep well hydrated through the fasting window. Any fluids need to be calorie free, so you can have water, black tea or coffee, herbal teas etc. I don't recommend any artificially sweetened drinks as they tend to trigger hunger and digestive juices – not what you need when there's no food coming. See below for more on ways to hydrate well and why adding a little salt to your water might help.

While we are digesting, the gut is not healing.

Aiming for a 12-hour no-calorie window most nights is a safe and sensible start to training your body to thrive without constant food hits. Begin to shift your last meal of the day a little earlier and if that's simply not practical, make it a lighter meal to help speed up digestion. Good management of your food and drink choices and food timings can make a big difference, giving your body and brain time to clean up, rest and renew. Remember, this is not going on while you are digesting food, which takes many hours.

Fasting interventions have been subject to deep scientific focus over the last few years that has revealed better outcomes for dementia, epilepsy, attention deficit disorders, multiple sclerosis and even Parkinson's and Alzheimer's disease, as well as depressive and anxiety disorders. One of the main hypotheses for these benefits is that fasting reduces inflammation through various mechanisms – as we saw in Chapter Four, lower inflammation is fundamental to a happy body and brain. With little to no food in the system, the body can switch gear to mend, restore and regenerate, reducing inflammation. Moreover, with fasting comes improved blood glucose control and greater insulin sensitivity, which enables body fat to be burned for fuel. That allows ketone production to begin, and ketones are the fast and clean fat-based fuel source that the brain loves to use (go back to Chapter Two for the benefits of supplying your brain with ketones).

When we eat less or less often, we enable body fat to be used as fuel in the form of ketones.

Regular fasting helps your hormone communication systems to become more finessed, allowing for better metabolic and nervous system regulation. Meanwhile the gut lining is cleaned up and the gut microbes are refreshing and renewing, preparing for the next eating window.

Furthermore, as brain scanning equipment has grown more sophisticated it has become evident that our brains possess an extraordinary ability to self-clean and heal. Improvements in the structure of the brain are seen when its cleaning systems are regularly activated. This largely happens at night, making good-quality sleep yet another must for a happy brain. Key to getting good sleep is to minimise digestive activity at night. If your stomach and the upper section of the small intestine are busy trying to break down and digest food, your body is biochemically unable to activate the deep, restorative sleep where brain cleaning occurs. You might fall asleep in a post-feast stupor, but that is not the same as achieving quality sleep.

Fasting can also help people reclaim a sense of structure and control over their eating patterns. Chaotic, compulsive eating habits and poor food choices are commonly experienced by those who are depressed and anxious, further adding to feelings of overwhelm and negativity. Having a positive plan around eating times and fasting times can bring about psychological as well as physical benefits.

It's very clear – having periods of time when we are not consuming food offers a potent combination of health benefits that translates to a happier brain.

N.B.: Those who are very underweight, breastfeeding mums and pregnant women should seek professional advice before undertaking any kind of fasting.

Fasting methods

There are various different methods and timings for fasting, so experiment with which one suits you best.

The 12/3 method has been researched by one of the leading experts in neurodegenerative diseases, Dr Dale Bredesen, and is part of his comprehensive protocol for Alzheimer's. It requires leaving at least 12 hours of no calories from the last to the first meal and having a 3-hour window from the last calories to bedtime to ensure good-quality sleep. [41] If you have been a constant grazer and late-night eater for much of your life, simply aim to stop eating at least 1 hour before bed and gradually build up to 3 hours.

This form of time-restricted eating is becoming increasingly accepted as a safe and sensible approach for many health conditions. The 12/3 approach is achievable for most people much of the time and it's a really great place to start your fasting explorations. There are numerous ways to achieve 12/3 without having to change too much about the rhythm of how you and your family live. Eat dinner earlier, have breakfast a little later and 12 hours should be easily achievable.

If 12/3 feels manageable, then you can begin to extend your 12-hour fasting window to 13 or 14 hours a few nights a week and see how you feel. For some people sleep, mood and energy all measurably improve, for others there can be limited if any benefit to a longer fasting window. Every body is unique and there are always so many factors at play, so it is important not to see this as an absolute without which your mental health will never improve. It's only one strategy among many that might be helpful for you. Be curious and open to what your unique body and brain respond best to.

16:8 is a popular fasting protocol and is suitable for many people, but not all. This means you eat and drink all calories, solids and liquids, within an 8-hour window. When you choose to have that eating window is up to you. It might be that having breakfast at 10 am and finishing dinner by 6 pm works well for you and your family. Some people simply don't feel like eating in the morning, so breaking their fast (having breakfast) at midday and finishing dinner by 8 pm is a comfortable and easy fit.

You can build up to a 16-hour fasting window if you are managing 12 and then 14 hours easily. These things are rarely absolute or linear, meaning some days you might easily manage 16 hours whereas the next day you know you need to eat after 12 hours. That's absolutely fine – it's important to honour your innate sense of what feels right while your body is getting used to the changes you are making. Exercise, your menstrual cycle, sleep quality and many other variables will change how long your body manages without food. Your brain is a hungry organ and some days it will demand more fuel more quickly than others.

Most people find their rhythm after a few months. Studies looking at the efficacy of 16:8 have found that just 2 days a week of a 16:8 protocol is enough to be beneficial.

5:2 is an alternative way of giving your body a digestive holiday. Rather than reducing the eating window, the focus is on reducing your intake. The late Michael Mosley, a well-known TV doctor and author, made this concept popular. It refers to 5 days of 'normal' eating with 2 days a week of reduced-calorie eating. When you reduce the amount of food you put through your system, you complete the process of digestion more quickly and healing can begin.

This protocol recommends around 800 calories on fasting days, considered a third of an adult's average intake. The calories can be consumed in one large meal or several small meals. Aim for two non-consecutive fasting days a week.

Midnight hunger

If you have poor blood glucose management you might find that fasting causes you to wake at night feeling hungry. It is not uncommon for people to wake in the small hours with a pounding heart as adrenaline surges due to low blood sugar levels. If you aren't able to sleep without midnight snacking, it's an indication that you have issues with your ability to burn fat. It could be insulin resistance, thyroid hormone irregularities or a combination of metabolic factors that keep your fat cells locked up at night instead of releasing their energy to fuel your overnight fast.

We require a surprisingly large amount of energy at night to perform all the healing and restoration that goes on during sleep. If your body cannot access the fuel in your fat stores due to elevated fasting insulin coming from chronic overstimulation of your blood glucose (this takes years for most people), inhibiting fat burning, your body will be forced to charge up your blood sugar with the help of a serious dose of stress hormones. It does this to ensure there is fuel in the system to keep everything ticking over properly while you sleep, but ironically it wakes you and keeps you awake. If this is your experience, gradually start to reduce the sugars and refined grains in your diet, and focus more on high-fibre foods, healthy fats and protein (see Chapter Six). As your insulin resistance improves, your body should adjust to managing your fat-burning systems better.

Again, don't push yourself too hard too quickly with these changes. See getting sleep as a priority over extending your fasting window. This is a process, something to work towards. If you find after a while that you don't respond well to these changes, you may want to get your thyroid, glucose and insulin levels checked to ensure there are no underlying endocrinological issues.

Postbiotics: The power of the 3Fs combined

Here's the big news. What results from combining the 3Fs is fascinating. When you feed your good gut microbes their favourite fuel source (prebiotic Fibre and polyphenols), top them up with live Fermented foods (probiotics) and then allow all that gut bug nourishment to work its magic with regular

Fasting windows, some pretty astounding happy brain magic takes place: it produces postbiotics or short-chain fatty acids (SCFAs). These (which you may remember from Chapter Four) are by-products made when our good gut microbes are thriving. The three main SCFAs, acetate, propionate and especially butyrate, have been well studied for their health benefits.

Prebiotics (fibre) feed probiotics (gut microbes) to make postbiotics (SCFAs).

Butyrate, also known as butyric acid, is the main fuel source of colonocytes, the cells that line the colon. These cells use butyrate to keep the colon healthy, greatly reducing the risk of colon cancer and other diseases of the large intestine. In return, the healthy environment that butyrate creates is a great host for the trillions of good gut microbes in our gut microbiome – it's a win–win. And it gets better: butyrate helps heal and seal the wall of the small intestine and the delicate blood–brain barrier. Further, if we have enough good gut bugs making butyrate, any excess butyrate above what the intestinal wall needs is passed around the body, providing potent antioxidant and anti-inflammatory effects, helping to reduce the oxidative and inflammatory damage known to directly affect mental health.

Increased butyrate to the brain provides better management of our neurochemistry, specifically serotonin and dopamine.

Butyrate directly influences the production of a growth factor made in the brain that maintains healthy neurotransmitter levels and gut–brain communication. This growth factor, BDNF (brain-derived neurotrophic factor, as also discussed in Chapter Four), is a core brain nutrient for neuroregeneration, balance and neuroplasticity, meaning the capacity to rewire and reprogram the brain to be healthier and happier. It helps the brain remain flexible, which is important for learning new skills, retaining information, balancing brain chemistry and optimising brain health in general. As BDNF levels increase thanks to the presence of butyrate, depression tends to improve. [42] The reverse can happen too:

> *An individual who does not consume enough fibre ... may experience a decrease in butyrate-producing bacteria ... leading to stress and inflammation and, potentially, symptoms of depression.* [43]

There are many other benefits of butyrate:

- The small intestine, where we absorb nutrients from food, has a mucous lining that is replaced every 3–4 days. The cells in the small intestine use butyrate to fuel this high turnover, keeping the small intestinal barrier healthy. That greatly helps in the prevention of leaky gut, a state of hyper-permeability where food particles and pathogens that should be kept in the gut can leak into the bloodstream causing immune irregularities, inflammation and many other health issues (see Chapter Three for more on this).
- Butyrate helps protect our cells from damage caused by oxidative stress. The main way it does this is by increasing levels of glutathione, known as the master antioxidant, which is made within our cells to protect them from free radical damage. [44]
- Butyrate influences our immune system in numerous ways, helping with its complex regulation.
- Butyrate enhances vagal tone when passing from the gut to the brain, improving our ability to recover from stress and trauma [45] (see Chapter Four for more on the vagus nerve).
- Butyrate has hormone-balancing effects that help with

obesity and type 2 diabetes. It works by increasing the release of the gut hormone GLP-1, which has had a lot of press coverage lately due to the popularity of the weight-loss drugs Ozempic and Wegovy. Such a drug and butyrate both work to increase GLP-1, which improves insulin sensitivity and appetite regulation. [46]

- Studies have shown better cholesterol management with increased butyrate production. [47]

There are specific strains of gut microbes that are prolific butyrate producers and certain foods and fibres that are especially supportive of this critical process. As most of us don't know which microbes we have or which type of fibre they are partial to, it's best to hedge our bets and eat according to the 3Fs. So get going on upping your Fibre, trying out some Fermented foods and Fast by reducing your eating window, at least by a little. These changes alone could get your happy brain action plan off to a great start.

CHAPTER SIX
Happy Brain Food Day to Day

As you have seen already in this book, what we eat directly and indirectly influences every part of our body and brain. Food is not just about energy (calories) or nutrients, like vitamins and minerals, it provides information and intelligence throughout the body. What we eat determines what our body does on a cellular level. Cells communicate with other cells, which then affects the function of our nerves, muscles, organs, hormones and immune system, all of which influence the brain. Eat well and our body works better – it's really that simple.

What eating well means for each one of us gets more complicated when we consider genetics, religious practices, social expectations, allergies, food sensitivities, and ethical and personal preferences. How we eat as well as what we eat is also important to consider. This chapter outlines some core principles of what and how to eat that promote a happy brain.

What is a healthy human diet?

This is a widely debated, often disagreed upon question. However, evolutionary science is generally united, due to fossilised evidence, that early man has been eating meat and bone marrow, as well as plant matter, for at least 2 ½ million years [48]. Human beings are omnivores, meaning our digestive tract, from mouth to anus, has evolved over millennia for the digestion of plants and animal products. In eating both plants and animal source foods, the human body and brain can get all essential nutrients required for cellular function to occur optimally. This then raises the question, if someone is choosing not to consume any animal products, are they able to thrive? This is where many disagreements occur, but it is factually correct that an entirely plant-based diet cannot adequately provide every nutrient the body needs. This is in part because some essential nutrients simply do not exist in plants, while there is the added complication that some people, due to genetics and their specific gut microbiome, cannot utilise certain nutrients in the plant form, which is often less bioavailable than the equivalent nutrient in animal form.

If you, or someone you know, is struggling with their mental health and are choosing to be 100% plant-based, please, at least consider, that maybe a plant-only diet is not optimal for your brain to be happy. As a minimum, you must supplement with key brain-supporting nutrients like vitamin B_{12}, likely vitamin D, iron, zinc, and the long-chain forms of omega 3, EPA and DHA. As hard as it might be, perhaps experiment with introducing some nutrient-rich animal foods, eggs are a fantastic place to start, and see how you feel. Animal foods, for some, are essential, I know – my body and brain were not able to thrive and be happy on a vegan diet, however hard I tried.

This isn't a diet that will come to an end once you feel better. A happy, healthy brain relies on a happy, healthy digestive system and your digestive system responds to every meal you eat. Of course you can let loose now and again, but if you can get to a place where roughly 80% of the time you are including happy brain foods and avoiding unhappy brain foods, your body and brain will be able to function in a healthier, happier way throughout your life.

So, what shall we eat?

Think fibre, ferments, protein and fats and you're covered!

The happy brain plate

In Chapter Five I said that a good estimate for the amount of fibre to eat was to fill half your plate with fibre-rich foods. To give you a clearer idea of what that means in practice, here's a more detailed example, but keep in mind that foods are rarely just one thing – pulses, for example, have some protein and are fibre rich as well as being starchy and nutritious, and avocado has great fibre and healthy fats. So this is simply a guide to help you create plates of food that cover all the bases:

- ⅓ (work up to closer to ½) a variety of low starch (low sugar) plant foods (mixed colourful salad, avocado, green beans, broccoli etc.) + some fermented veggies like sauerkraut or kimchi
- ⅓ protein-rich foods (fish, meat, eggs, fermented dairy, tofu or other fermented soy / high quality plant-protein)
- ⅙ - ⅓ nutrient-rich starchy foods (sweet potatoes, squash, quinoa, pulses frozen peas). This is optional. For those aiming for more a ketogenic protocol, replace these foods for more fats and fattier protein sources)
- Topped off with some healthy fats (olive oil dressing, pumpkin seeds, walnuts, avocado slices) and / or spices, toppings (or treats)

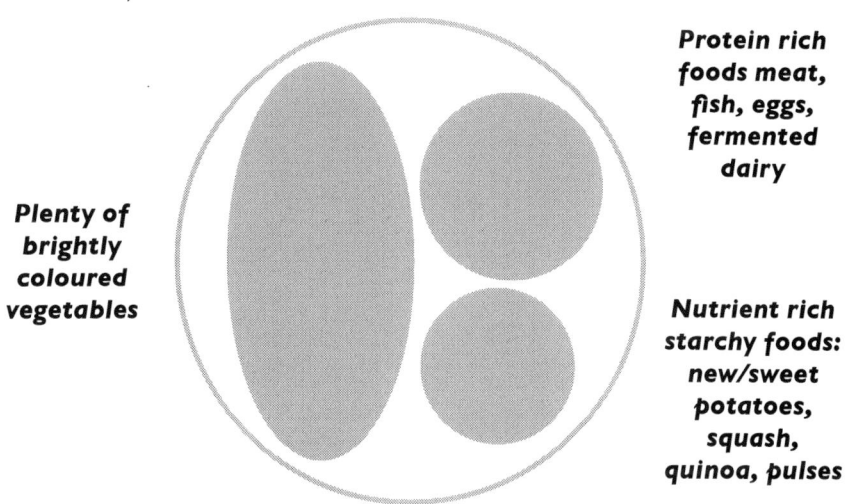

Plenty of brightly coloured vegetables

Protein rich foods meat, fish, eggs, fermented dairy

Nutrient rich starchy foods: new/sweet potatoes, squash, quinoa, pulses

Let's look at each of these groups in turn.

Fibre-rich plant foods

We saw in Chapter Five that we need fibre to feed our happy gut microbes, but wholesome plant foods contain more than that. There is a highly complex range of nutrients and natural plant compounds that humans evolved to consume that are lacking in highly processed foods. The more a food resembles how it looks in nature, the better. Moreover, many of the preservatives, emulsifiers and other additives found in highly processed foods can derail our gut microbes and their ability to communicate around the body and up to the brain. This can drive desperate food cravings and compulsive over-eating, or conversely loss of appetite and interest in food.

Healthier swaps include:

- A whole orange rather than orange juice
- Whole almonds rather than almond butter, almond flour or almond milk
- Whole jumbo oats rather than instant porridge pots or oat milk
- Butter rather than vegetable spread
- Boiled or oven-roasted potatoes rather than instant mash or potato-based snacks
- Whole beans and lentils rather than a processed veggie burger or lentil crisps

Aim to include on your plate vegetables, fruits, beans, lentils, nuts and seeds of as many types as possible. Think of the colours of the rainbow and lots of different foods rather than lots of the same. A wide, diverse range of plant foods is essential for a healthy gut microbiome because it provides different kinds of fibre for our gut microbes.

Consider signing up for a local veg box or use one of the national food delivery services that supply seasonal fresh produce, preferably locally grown. They are often competitively priced and are a great way to get you and your family eating a wider range of fresh veggies.

A good challenge is to try at least once a week to buy a vegetable you don't usually eat. Look up how to cook it if you need to. Then if you like it, add it to your weekly shop.

Don't forget the freezer aisle. Frozen peas are fibre rich and packed full of vitamins and minerals, and bags of mixed frozen vegetables are a great option too.

Because fruit contains sugar and sugar can feed microbes that are not so happy brain friendly, you want to limit your fruit intake and focus more on veggies. Remember 5:2 a day – 5 portions of vegetables (including salad) and 2 portions of fruit. Also combine fruit with other foods to balance out the sugars. Berries or a kiwi fruit with live natural yogurt, nuts and seeds is a fabulous fibre-rich combo, and half a sliced apple with a little mature cheese or a handful of nuts makes for a great balanced snack. Seasonal fruits are always a better option than those shipped halfway around the world and frozen berries are a great staple during the winter months.

Beans and lentils, commonly referred to as pulses, are nutrient rich and have really significant levels of fibre, including resistant starch, which you may recall from Chapter Five is a favourite fuel for your happy gut bugs. Pulses are extremely cheap, especially if you buy them dried, but do bear in mind that dried beans require some careful soaking and cooking otherwise they can be indigestible and in the case of red kidney beans actually quite toxic, so you may prefer tinned or jarred instead. They're lovely added to salads, soups and stews. Mix some butter beans or chickpeas through a tray of roasted veg along with some feta cheese or chorizo chunks and a generous sprinkling of freshly chopped parsley for a hearty, balanced and gut-nourishing dish.

When beans and seeds are soaked and then sprouted they become significantly more nutritious and far more digestible. Just as a seed or bean is breaking open and growing its first sprout, the nourishment is readily available to be digested. Simply soak in water a range of seeds and legumes (easy ones are mung beans, green lentils and sunflower seeds) in a glass jar for at least 12 hours. Drain and then leave at room temperature, out of direct sunlight, for a few days until you see shoots start to appear. You must rinse and drain daily. Once they have sprouted, eat them in salads with olive oil. They will keep in the fridge for a few days. You can use a sprouting jar that has a draining lid incorporated into it, but that is not a necessity.

Nuts and seeds come in many forms and again, diversity is key. They are impressively nutrient dense, containing all the nutrients required to grow a fully fledged plant, so when we eat nuts and seeds we benefit by getting great fats, protein and fibre along with a multitude of vitamins, minerals and phytochemicals.

If you find nuts or seeds indigestible (are you seeing bits in your poop?) then try soaking them in water overnight. This greatly helps you break down and absorb the many nutrients while providing 'swollen', water-soaked fibre to fuel your gut bugs. Flax and chia seeds should always be soaked to provide your digestive system and your microbes with the gloopy mucilage that comes from doing this. It also means you are more likely to digest and absorb all the nutrients in chia and flax rather than pooping them out in the same form they went in.

My happy gut smoothie uses soaked flax and chia seeds and is an easy way to add a variety of nutrients into your day. It's a great combination of good fats, protein and a range of fibres and polyphenols. Have it in place of breakfast or add to a breakfast bowl of 2 tablespoons of whole oats, flax and chia seeds soaked overnight, topped with live natural yogurt. Alternatively, have your super-smoothie along with an egg dish to create a more substantial breakfast or brunch.

Stephanie J's Happy Gut Smoothie

Use a wide range of the ingredients below to ensure your smoothie contains plenty of good fat, fibre and protein. It isn't meant to taste sweet, but it should taste delicious. As your tastebuds adjust to being bludgeoned less often with sugar, you will enjoy more bitter and savoury flavours. Meanwhile, adding a little raw honey or natural sweetener like stevia or monk fruit powder can help.

Ingredients
- 1 handful of dark berries (frozen mixed summer berries are great for this)
- 2 tablespoons of soaked flax and chia seeds (with the soaking liquid)
- 2 tablespoons of sugar-free coconut or dairy kefir (highly fermented drink)
- 2 heaped teaspoons of raw cacao powder (lots of polyphenols, fibre and magnesium)
- 1 heaped teaspoon of maca powder (lovely vanilla flavour and great for hormones and reducing stress levels)
- 1 teaspoon of matcha green tea powder (superfood for gut microbes and brain health)
- 1 teaspoon of Ceylon cinnamon (great for blood glucose management)
- 1 teaspoon of black cumin seed oil (an all-round superfood – see the next section)
- 1 very fresh raw egg (optional)
- 1 teaspoon of a prebiotic fibre supplement (optional – see Chapter Eight)
- 20 g (usually 2 scoops) of a good-quality protein powder such as whey isolate, bone broth powder or hemp to ensure you get adequate protein. Especially important if you plan to have the smoothie after a tough workout and/or are breaking a

- longer fast
- A shot of espresso if you're having it as a morning pre-workout smoothie

Add water to get the right consistency.

Befriend bitter foods

Consuming bitter herbs (bitters) or digestifs used to be a traditional pre-meal practice and still is in some countries. Bitter flavours help stimulate saliva and digestive signalling, enhancing the absorption of nutrients from your meals. For a pre-meal tincture, add a few drops of digestive bitters to a little water, swill this around your mouth and swallow it shortly before you start to eat. This is especially helpful for people who suffer with bloating, burping, feeling tired and heavy after eating or are prone to reflux issues.

Commercially available digestive bitters, often termed 'Swedish bitters', contain herbs such as gentian, dandelion, thistle and angelica that you're not likely to be including in your diet. These bitter-tasting herbs are distilled in alcohol to extract their healthful properties. You can also make your own teas and tinctures if you're so inclined. If you don't have access to digestive bitters, a tablespoon of apple cider vinegar in around 80–100 ml of water is a great alternative.

Also aim to include a few bitter leaves with your meals, such as chicory/endive, radicchio, rocket and watercress. Not only are these great for revving up your digestive juices, they contain prebiotic fibre and polyphenols, helping to fuel your happy gut bugs.

Experiment with other bitter foods and flavours:

- Turmeric is a superstar bitter spice, as are saffron and paprika.
- The stems of romaine and little gem lettuce are deliciously

- bitter and extremely happy- gut friendly, so don't throw them away. Finely slice the stems and add them to your salad along with the lettuce leaves.
- The brassica family – broccoli, cabbage, cauliflower and Brussel sprouts – contain some bitter compounds, although sadly these foods are being engineered to have less bitterness and more sweetness.
- Eat the darkest chocolate you can tolerate and nudge up the percentage of cocoa solids as time goes by to keep training your taste buds away from wanting something sweet to loving something bitter. Cacao, the raw cocoa bean, is teeming with healthy bitter polyphenols.
- Teas of all colours – 'builder's' (black) tea, green tea (especially Matcha), white tea – as well as good-quality coffee are polyphenol rich.

Mix and match these bitter, health-giving foods to give your gut and brain a boost on a regular basis.

Black seed oil

Black (cumin) seed oil is another bitter food that is anti-inflammatory and an all-round health booster. You may not be familiar with it, yet it's been used for over 1000 years in some countries and has been the subject of several scientific studies. An Islamic hadith said the 'blessed seed' was 'healing for all diseases except death'. [49] It can be taken in spoonfuls like a medicine or used in dressings or smoothies.

Research into the effects of black seed oil show clinically significant improvements in levels of anxiety and depression as well as memory impairment, neurodegeneration and pain. It is a complex oil with many active compounds, so it is hard to establish how and why these improvements are seen. Certainly there are anti-inflammatory benefits and gut-friendly polyphenols, which are what give black seed oil its bitter taste. Some of the health effects that have been shown include the following:

- An increase in the production of L-tryptophan, the precursor ingredient to serotonin and melatonin, was found over one four-week trial using 500 mg of black seed oil daily, and the 14–17-year-old males involved showed *'significant mood improvement, decreased anxiety, and a boost in cognition'*. [50]
- Another study was conducted in 2021 at military hospitals in Tehran on 52 male patients with major depressive disorder taking antidepressants. Half of the men were given 1000 mg of black seed oil for 10 weeks, the other half were given a placebo. The group taking the oil scored far lower on the, Anxiety, and Stress Scale-21 Items (DASS-21) compared to the placebo group and there was an increase in serum BDNF (see Chapters Four and Five). [51]
- Some studies suggest that black seed oil can partially regenerate cells in the pancreas that produce insulin, hence both type 1 and type 2 diabetics might benefit. It also acts in the same way as the most readily prescribed drug for type 2 diabetes, metformin. (Take your doctor's advice before making any changes to your medication.)
- A compound in black seed oil called thymoquinone has been shown to be effective against multiple strains of the hospital-acquired bug MRSA. Thymoquinone is an antioxidant, anti-inflammatory, anti-viral, anti-microbial, immune system modulator and anti-coagulant.
- Black seed oil has multiple anti-cancer properties: restricting increase in the growth of new blood vessels to a tumour (anti-angiogenesis); preventing metastasis or the spreading of cancer to other areas; triggering cell death in cancer (something that healthy cells know to do if they are damaged or malfunctioning, but cancer cells are not capable of); and enhancing the efficacy of chemotherapy while reducing side effects.

- Black seed oil offers protection and detoxification support to the liver.
- Black seed oil helps to feed the beneficial gut microbes while helping to rid the digestive tract of pathogenic and parasitic overgrowth.
- Black seed oil can help with systemic inflammation and seems to be helpful with many respiratory issues.

Fermented foods

We looked at these in depth in Chapter Five as the second of the 3Fs. These vibrant, living foods are extremely helpful for a happy gut and brain and many are surprisingly easy to make for little cost. The fermented foods and drinks to be consumed on a regular basis to support your gut–brain axis are:

- Fermented vegetables: sauerkraut, kimchi or any mix of brined and fermented veggies
- Fermented, unsweetened dairy like live yogurt, dairy kefir, mature cheese
- Raw apple cider vinegar
- Water kefir, coconut kefir and kombucha
- Fermented soy: miso, natto, fermented tofu
- Traditional cured meats: kabanos, chorizo, salami, prosciutto
- Traditionally brined olives and gherkins

N.B.: Pickles in vinegar are not the same as fermented veggies. Fermented vegetables taste sour due to the lactic acid that is naturally produced through the fermentation process. Vinegary foods are sour because of the acetic acid in the vinegar they have been soaked in. Pickles in vinegar do not have the same beneficial microbes as fermented foods.

Some people can find traditionally fermented foods challenging at first due to their sour flavour. Sourness signifies fermentation and that's a good thing. Start with small amounts, hide them in other foods to dilute the flavour (but don't heat them) and over time you might find them really enjoyable. The more you stay away from sweet foods, the more quickly your palate will acclimatise to these sour flavours.

Aim to have some form of fermented food every day, even if it's a small spoonful of sauerkraut mixed through a salad or a dollop of live yogurt with your breakfast. Ideally mix them up to ensure a wide range of microbes, as each type of fermented food contains different beneficial bacteria, helping to top up your gut microbes faster than they are being killed off by other aspects of your diet.

Protein-rich foods

Having plenty of colourful, fibre-rich and fermented foods is all very well, but they don't constitute a complete and balanced diet. You need protein too, as well as fat (which we'll look at next). How much and which types of protein are still hotly contested. For instance, vegans consider all animal products disastrous for human health and the health of the planet, while those who advocate the 'carnivore' diet view plant-based foods as toxic, indigestible and ruinous to the gut. I suspect there is a healthy and happy place for the human diet and the planet somewhere in the middle.

What is clear is that we all have different dietary requirements based on genetics, our gut microbiome and our lifestyle choices. As such, it's best to focus on what we do know from our understanding of evolutionary science and human nutritional requirements – and that is that humans are adaptable omnivores.

What is an absolute fact is that protein – or rather amino acids, which is what protein is broken down into through the process of good digestion – is fundamental to human life. Without the nine essential amino acids that come from certain forms of protein, our body and brain simply cannot function. These nine essential amino acids link up with each other in different combinations and lengths to form further amino acids. In total the human body requires 20 amino acids to make brain chemicals; bone and muscle tissue; a healthy gut lining; skin, hair and nail cells; blood cells; hormone and immune cells; and the 75,000+ enzymes that allow all these bodily processes to work – all of these require amino acids. Our cells are continuously being created and broken down, and getting adequate protein and digesting it well are essential to keep these systems well supplied.

For the body to be able to use protein of any kind requires good protein digestion, which takes place largely in the stomach, right at the top of the digestive system. Chewing well, eating in a calm and focused state and savouring your food greatly improve the process of breaking down your food proteins into the much-needed individual amino acids. Once the stomach has churned up your proteins with lots of stomach acid and protein-digesting enzymes, the amino acids are made available to be absorbed into your bloodstream, where they are sent around the body to mend, restore, build and balance.

Good mental health requires good protein digestion

Good mental health requires a ready supply of well-digested protein to provide the intricate balance of amino acids that is the foundation to happy brain chemistry. But the body cannot digest protein into amino acids without adequate stomach acid.

Causes of low stomach acid include:

Chronic stress
Acid-blocking medications
Lack of certain nutrients like zinc and B vitamins
Having a poorly functioning vagus nerve
Smoking
Alcohol
Eating in a rushed and distracted state

> *Eating highly processed foods that need very little if any chewing*
> *Living on a very low-protein diet*
>
> *All of these suppress stomach acid production, reducing the availability of amino acids for the manufacture of happy brain chemistry.*

Protein fills us up quickly and keeps us feeling satisfied for long periods of time. This can help manage appetite, cravings, over-eating and ultimately our weight. If we have adequate amounts of good-quality protein every time we eat, our brain receives a signal through our nutrient-sensing system that we have been well nourished. This sense of being replete and truly satiated is important if we are to avoid cravings and the drive to snack and over-consume, which can lead to poor food choices and excess body fat, driving a poorly balanced, inflamed and unhappy brain. Another reason protein is so helpful is that it helps to stabilise our blood glucose levels, which is also important for a happy brain.

Animal-based protein

You can be an animal lover and you can care deeply about the environment while eating animal products. If they are sourced well and prepared and eaten with care, animal products are an integral part of a happy brain diet. Meat, fish, seafood, eggs and dairy contain all nine essential amino acids and mostly offer a well-balanced combination. Animal proteins are also more bio-available than plant proteins, meaning the protein is more readily digested, requiring less volume of the protein-rich food to meet our nutrient needs.

Having a little (or a lot if you want) of some animal-based foods with most or all of your meals is a quick and simple way of ensuring you are getting the building blocks your body needs along with those critical brain-friendly nutrients iron, zinc, omega 3 fatty acids (oily fish and meat from grass-fed animals – more on these in the healthy fats section), vitamin B_{12}, vitamin D and ready-formed vitamin A (find out about vitamins in Chapter Eight).

Here are some quick and simple ways to nudge up your protein intake:

- A couple of hard-boiled eggs chopped up in a salad along with a generous grating of Parmesan cheese or some tinned tuna or sardines
- Feta cheese sprinkled over roasted veg
- Prawns in a stir-fry or with lentil pasta
- A fish fillet (not in batter or breadcrumbs) with veggies and an avocado and sauerkraut salad
- Roasted chicken thighs with a range of veg or salads
- A burger with a high meat content on a large, garlicky Portobello mushroom
- Sausages with a high meat content and cheesy cauliflower and broccoli mash

It doesn't have to be complicated or expensive to create a well-balanced and nourishing meal. Think of different ways to add a wider range of ingredients and lots of different vegetables alongside a source of protein. To help make animal protein go further, you can include plant sources such as butter beans mixed in with roasted vegetables, or a chickpea dip (hummus) and a sprinkling of nuts and seeds in your salad. Lentils are lovely added to minced meat dishes and a cheese, rocket and mushroom omelette is a quick, easy breakfast, lunch or light supper option that ticks all the boxes.

Many people find they feel a lot better when they include more protein in their meals. At first it can be subtle, but over time you might find you recover more quickly from exercise and see the benefits more readily. Your hair, skin and nails might improve while your energy levels and appetite become more balanced. Most importantly, you might begin to struggle less with unstable moods, anxious thoughts and an unhappy brain.

As with food of any kind, having animal protein in a minimally processed form is best. This means rather than products that contain lots of additional ingredients, go for plain cuts of meat and fish or whole eggs and combine them with other foods to create wholesome meals. Vary your choices throughout the week, having some fish, seafood, meat, poultry, eggs, natural yogurt or cheese with each meal, or a generous source of plant protein (see the section below).

Look at the ingredients list

Don't trust what's on the front of the packaging of any processed food, even if it is promoted as healthy or high in protein. The pictures and descriptions can be very misleading. For example, a well-known brand of meat pie contains only 13% beef, providing only 9 g of protein, just a little more than the protein in one large egg. With the meat content of the meat pie being so low, the dish inevitably includes many other ingredients that are not especially nourishing, including refined grains and oils, sugar, emulsifiers and colourings. This information is readily available on the back of the packet, so it's worth taking an extra few seconds to read the ingredients list to see what you're actually buying. Nutritional data is required on all packaged foods, and that will tell you how much protein there is.

A typical ready-made meat pie

Typical Values	As Sold 100 g Provides:	Per Pie Provides:
Energy – kJ	1253 kJ	1922 kJ
– kcal	300 kcal	460 kcal
Fat	17 g	26 g
– of which Saturates	7.6 g	12 g
Carbohydrate	30 g	46 g
– of which Sugars	0.8 g	1.2 g
Fibre	2.1 g	3.3 g
Protein	5.7 g	8.9 g
Salt	0.59 g	0.91 g

> Ingredients
> Flour (**Wheat**, Maize), Water, Minced Beef (13%), Pork Lard, Potato (6%), Brown Ale (3%) (**Barley, Wheat**), Onion, Starch (Modified Maize, Maize), **Barley** Fibre, Beef Stock (Beef Stock, Sugar, Carrot Juice Concentrate, Onion Concentrate, Tomato Paste), **Celery** Salt (Salt, **Celery** Extract, Celery Seed Oil), Salt, Glucose Syrup, **Barley** Malt Extract, Pea Protein, Calcium Carbonate, Tomato Powder, Onion Powder, Cocoa Powder, Rapeseed Oil, Maltodextrin, Dextrose, Black Pepper, Dried Rosemary, Niacin, Iron, Thiamine

Another example is breaded chicken pieces, which contain a lot more than just chicken and breadcrumbs. With a little extra effort and probably for less money you can buy some plain chicken pieces, dip them in egg, coat them in breadcrumbs whizzed up in a food processor (or nut flour) and oven roast with a range of vegetables. That gives you a delicious and nutritious meal without the preservatives, sugar and other ingredients in the processed variety.

Plant-based protein

Plenty of plant foods contain some protein – beans, lentils, soy, nuts and seeds; even grains like oats and rice contain a little protein. Mung beans have the highest level of protein of all pulses, three times that of red lentils. Quinoa (a pseudo-grain) has more than twice the protein content of rice by weight. However, no plant contains good levels of all the nine essential amino acids, although fermented soy products such as natto, tempeh and fermented tofu come close. So it's essential that anyone eating an exclusively plant-based diet carefully combines different plant-based proteins to avoid deficiencies of single amino acids.

Because plants have low levels of amino acids compared to animal foods, it's also necessary to eat a large volume of them to get sufficient protein for all our physiological needs. This is a great way to consume lots of fibre, but many people struggle with the sheer amount they have to eat, and bloating and gut irritation are common complaints due to the volume of fibrous plants being consumed. Some people are better at digesting and extracting the protein from plant-based foods than others. This is dependent on their gut microbial families, their genetics and their dietary and medical history, which is why some people can function much better than others on plant-only proteins.

Amino acids are not held in reserve within the body even though they're essential to all critical functions, so we need to provide sufficient amounts of them every day. Be sensitive to your personal needs. If you choose to eat an exclusively plant-based diet and your body and brain are happy, energised and resilient, then you are likely meeting all your amino acid needs. If you are not optimally well, then maybe consider introducing some carefully selected animal products to top up your essential amino acid balance, such as local free-range eggs or some oily wild fish like sardines.

The missing link in plant proteins

Lysine is an essential amino acid that is especially hard to get enough of through exclusively plant-based proteins. It is involved in the release of serotonin and management of the stress hormone cortisol. A lack of lysine can therefore affect sleep and mood, trigger anxiety and exacerbate depression. Soy is the best non-animal source of lysine, but few people eat enough of it to get adequate amounts. Sardines, eggs, Parmesan cheese and free-range chicken are all great additions, even in small amounts, to balance the amino acids in a plant-based dish and provide plenty of lysine.

If you choose not to eat any animal products, it is critical you get your nutrient status tested to ensure your diet is providing adequate amino acids, in particular lysine, carnitine and tryptophan, the main ingredient of serotonin, as well as other nutrients typically lacking in plant foods: iron, zinc, omega 3 fatty acids, vitamin B_{12}, vitamin D and vitamin A (not beta-carotene – this is found in plant foods and can be converted to true vitamin A, but it is not a reliable source for everyone as some people are poor converters.

Beta-carotene does not provide the same benefits as fully formed vitamin A). It is really challenging, some experts say impossible, to meet all these requirements without supplementing. Many people find their mental health improves rapidly and substantially once they supplement well or return to eating animal-based products at least occasionally.

Eating large amounts of plant-based foods can also be challenging for blood glucose balance. Plant-based diets invariably include lots of grains, starchy vegetables and fruit, all of which can certainly be part of a healthy diet, but in large quantities can lead to elevated blood glucose. Since chronic excess glucose is known to be a problem in the brains of many people with mental health challenges, purely plant-based diets can be problematic for those with depression and anxiety.

If you would like to know more about the potential complications of mental health problems on a plant-based diet, look up the work of psychiatrist James Greenblatt, who has written many articles and given many interviews on this subject. [52]

How much protein is enough?

Eating more protein more regularly is not the same as eating a very high-protein diet – that is not what I'm recommending here. Sensible, well-researched recommendations for daily protein intake vary from 0.75 g to 2.2 g of protein per kg of body weight depending on your activity level and various complicated metrics. Such a wide range is not very helpful, so don't feel you need to be working out what your ideal intake of protein is. For many people and especially those who are grappling with mental health issues, this might well feel too taxing and confusing. If you do like to work these things out, there are many online resources to help you such as the app MyFitnessPal.

As a rough guide, 1.4–1.6 g of protein per kg of body weight per day, spread throughout the day, is a good start, more if you're very physically active. Body builders typically have at least 2.4 g of protein per kg of body weight per day — that's a lot of protein and is not required or recommended for most people. So as an example, a 70 kg person would require around 70 × 1.5 = 105 g of protein per day.

Here are some common foods and their protein values to give you a sense of what is required to hit around 100 g of protein a day (the exact values will vary according to the type and or brand). Notice how adding in small extras like pumpkin seeds or beans bumps up the levels nicely.

- 150 g of Greek yogurt (1 small pot) = 15 g
- 1 tablespoon of hemp protein powder = 5 g
- 2 heaped tablespoons of pumpkin seeds = 6 g
- 6 walnut halves = 4 g
- 25 g cheddar cheese or 2 heaped tablespoons of cottage cheese = 6 g
- 100 g or ¼ of an average block of tofu = 13 g
- 3 medium eggs = 18 g
- 1 tablespoon of peanut butter = 4 g
- Half a tin (200 g) of black beans or lentils (drained) = 6 g
- 1 medium chicken breast or beef burger (approx. 100 g) or 110 g tin of tuna (drained) = 24 g

Think about the meals you eat on a regular basis. If your plate or bowl is mostly or entirely made up of bread, rice, potatoes or pasta and veg, with little to no protein, play around with some of the ideas in that list to create a better balance. As you start to get a handle on protein you can look up recipes online or get a cookbook that incorporates higher-protein meals. Some great cookbooks are listed in the resources section at the end of the book.

Nutrient-rich starchy foods

These are what I call the beneficial carbs. They do have the potential to rev up blood glucose if eaten too often, in too high quantities or when highly refined, so the form matters and for some people these foods need to be limited or avoided in whatever form. This is all down to the individual's blood glucose and degree of insulin resistance. For many people, when these starchier foods are eaten in their whole form along with protein, healthy fats (see below) and a fibre-rich, low-starch carb, they are great filler-uppers while offering a wide range of nutrients plus prebiotic fibre and great convenience – pre-cooked pulses in tins or jars are a simple option. Aim for these foods to make up roughly 25% of your meals.

Beneficial carbs include:

- A small serving of new potatoes, sweet potatoes and parsnips – these are all high-starch veggies that can really spike blood glucose, large white potatoes being the worst culprit and sweet potatoes the best out of the three listed here. Ideally eat these after they have been cooked and cooled for at least six hours and then reheat or eat them cold, as this reduces the impact on blood glucose while increasing the benefit to your healthy gut microbes.
- Beans and lentils – no need to cook from scratch if time is tight. The beans and lentils pre-cooked in jars and tins are fantastic! Eating them in their whole form is best. They are lovely for adding bulk to soups, stews and salads, but crackers and pastas made from pulses are also good options and generally a healthier choice than those made from wheat.
- Squash/pumpkin – experiment with different types. All are great roasted or in soups.
- Quinoa, buckwheat and amaranth – known as pseudo-grains as they are not technically grains.
- Rye bread and crackers – some people are very sensitive to the gluten containing grains, wheat, rye and barley, which tend to cause bloating shortly after eating and can lead to rapid energy crashes. If this is not you, then sourdough bread or crackers made from wheat can be used sparingly,

but sourdough bread and crackers made from rye are better still. Rye grain is darker, more dense (so less easy to overeat) and is lower in gluten, higher in resistant starch and generally less inflammatory than wheat. Traditional pumpernickel bread is made from minimally processed rye grains and is great toasted, although it does take several dunks to get it crispy. Finn Crisp is a brand of sourdough rye crackers that have very few ingredients and are less processed than classics like Ryvita.

Healthy fats

As well as the essential amino acids that come from protein, there are essential fatty acids that come from the fats in our food. (Interestingly, there is no such thing as an essential carbohydrate – if we need glucose (sugar) we can make it in the body.) Our brain is made up of a lot of fat, our nerves and cells are coated in fat and many of our hormones and neurotransmitters are composed of fats.

Good-quality fats mean good-quality nerves, cells, hormones and brain chemistry.

For years fat has been vilified as the supposed cause of health issues including obesity and heart disease, but this has now largely been debunked. It is the source and quality of the fats we eat that matter, far more than the amount of fat. There is little conclusive evidence to support the idea that animal fats cause heart disease, whereas it is well established [53] that trans fats, the highly processed fats found in many packaged foods and now strictly regulated, and highly refined vegetable and seed oils, found throughout the food processing and fast-food industries, lack nutrients, are highly inflammatory and should be limited or avoided. This is especially true when processed fats and oils are combined with sugars and starches, as in biscuits, desserts, crisps and deep-fried foods. The sweet and fatty combo is deeply satisfying and can provide a momentary lift, but the potential upset to your gut microbes and mental health is much longer lasting.

Keep things simple and use the principle of the least processing possible. Fats and oils can become oxidised and turn rancid, rendering them not only unpleasant to taste and smell but highly toxic and inflammatory. The more a fat or oil has been processed, the more likely it is to have become spoiled. Moreover, some fats and oils tolerate light, heat and oxygen better than others.

Here's a list of the most gut- and brain-healthy fats and oils. All of these require minimal mechanical extraction and /or heat or solvents to be produced from their whole form.

For cooking:
- Extra virgin olive oil (for cooking at medium heat)
- Avocado oil (better than olive oil for higher temperatures)
- Butter (medium heat)
- Ghee (better than butter for higher temperatures)
- Extra virgin coconut oil (medium-high heat)
- Rendered fats from animals reared organically, such as lard, dripping/tallow or chicken/goose/duck fat (high heat)

For dressing salads or other foods:
- Extra virgin olive oil
- Cold-pressed black seed oil
- Avocado oil
- Nut oils (buy in very small amounts and keep in a cool, dark place to avoid spoiling)

Further sources of healthy fats are free-range, organic eggs (more specifically the yolks, which are enriched with omega 3 through the hens eating a natural healthy diet rather than grain-based feed), whole nuts and seeds, grass-fed meat and wild oily fish.

The intensive industrial processing required to extract standard seed and vegetable oils such as sunflower, rapeseed, corn and soybean oils results in aggressive inflammatory compounds being present when we come to consume them. This is especially true when these oils are repeatedly heated, as in deep-fat friers. Be very selective about buying any ready-made dressings and sauces because they often contain rapeseed or sunflower seed oil. Instead, make your own simple dressing that you can flavour with herbs of your choice.

Simple Happy-Brain Dressing

- 3 tablespoons of extra virgin olive oil
- 1 tablespoon of raw apple cider vinegar or lemon juice
- 1 teaspoon of mustard of your choice
- A little crushed garlic
- Freshly chopped parsley, mint, coriander, rosemary or basil
- 1 tablespoon of live natural yogurt or dairy kefir (optional)

Put all the ingredients in a clean jam jar and shake like crazy, or whizz them up in a blender.

Essential fatty acids

The two essential fatty acids that we need in order to function are omega 3 and omega 6. We cannot make them in the body, so we have to get them from food. They confer opposing benefits: omega 3 is highly anti-inflammatory, omega 6 is pro-inflammatory.

Omega 3 fatty acids are critical to healing, calming and balancing the brain. They are integral to our immune, hormone and neurological systems; they keep cell and blood vessel walls healthy; and they are also thought to help maintain a healthy gut and brain lining, preventing toxins escaping the gut and entering the brain. With all I have written about the dangers of inflammation to our mental well-being, you might think that omega 6 fatty acids being pro-inflammatory is not good. To a certain extent you'd be right, but it's all about the dose. Acute inflammation is life-saving to fight infection and heal wounds, and omega 6 is a critical part of that process. However, if we have too much it can lead to chronic inflammation within our cells, including in our brain. An excess of omega 6 can also block the uptake of omega 3, as both omega 6 and omega 3 enter our cells through the same doorway. If the door is blocked with lots of omega 6, the omega 3 can't get where it needs to go.

Omega 6 fatty acids are very easy to over-consume in the modern diet. Grains, nuts and seeds, vegetable and seed oils, grain-fed animals (like corn-fed chicken) and very many processed foods, ready meals and takeaway foods will have significant levels of omega 6. Consuming some omega 6–containing wholefoods such as whole sunflower seeds is not such a problem. It's the extraction and over-consumption of concentrated forms, such as sunflower oil, that is more concerning.

To sum up, sources of omega 6 fatty acids include:

- Seed and vegetable oils
- Deep-fried foods
- Fast foods
- Meat and eggs from corn (grain)-fed animals
- Corn-based snacks
- Peanuts/peanut butter
- Soy
- Almonds – whole and almond butter (almond milk has a negligible amount)
- Sunflower seeds

In contrast, it's really hard for most people to consume enough omega 3 fatty acids, found in oily fish such as sardines, mackerel, anchovies and wild (not farmed) salmon. We need to be eating several servings a week of these oily fish to get enough omega 3.

> **Omega 3 for a happy brain**
>
> *Research has shown that the higher a country's fish consumption the lower the incidence of depression, with the highest doses of omega 3 intake having the greatest overall effect.* [54] *This was found for those on antidepressants as well as those who were not.*

Many studies showing the benefit of omega 3 consumption to depressed patients use fish oil supplements at a dose of 2–4 g a day. To put this into perspective, you would only gain 1 g of omega 3 from eating three portions of oily fish a week. Therefore, supplementation is probably a good idea. Go to Chapter Eight for details on what to look for, as not all omega 3 supplements are equal.

Organic free-range eggs also provide a little omega 3, as does grass-fed meat. The stipulation of outdoor reared and grass fed is critical, as it is what the animal eats that determines whether or not you get omega 3 from eating them – you are what you eat ate! This also applies to farmed salmon, which don't have the beneficial omega 3 fats that come from wild salmon that eat algae and krill.

There are some omega 3 fats in chia and flax seeds and walnuts, but the levels and structure of these plant-based omegas are often inadequate and are poorly utilised by the body.

To sum up, sources of omega 3 fatty acids include:
- Sardines
- Mackerel
- Herring
- Wild salmon

- Anchovies
- Organic free-range eggs
- Chia and flax seeds
- Text BoxWalnuts

> **If we are over-consuming omega 6 and under-consuming omega 3, we are more prone to inflammation. Inflammation in the brain increases the likelihood of anxiety and depression.**

To help manage the critical balance between these essential fatty acids:

- Limit your intake of omega 6–rich oils by reducing or avoiding deep-fried foods, processed and packaged foods, and change the cooking oils you use at home for the healthier ones I listed earlier.
- Increase your omega 3 intake by consuming oily fish several times a week. Tinned sardines or mackerel in olive oil or spring water are good, easy and relatively cheap options. Fresh tuna and wild salmon are also good sources to have on occasion, although a rare treat for most people. Many supermarkets have frozen wild salmon fillets, which tend to be cheaper.
- Supplementation of omega 3 is an easy way to ensure you're meeting your requirement for these essential happy brain fats. There is more on supplements in Chapter Eight.

Hydration

No chapter on happy brain food would be complete without a nod to good hydration. This is absolutely not about downing large volumes of water to hit the often mentioned 3 litres a day (there is no scientific evidence to support this). However, your brain and body cannot self-regulate well if you are under-hydrating, so ensuring adequate fluids and fluid-filled foods throughout the day is important. Classic signs of dehydration are grogginess, brain fog, headaches, aches and pains, general fatigue and hunger pangs, which are often actually thirst signals.

If your body is dehydrated, this is just one more high-alert alarm bell that will be jangling your nervous system, triggering stress hormones and preventing vagus nerve activation. That is going to contribute to an unhappy brain on many levels. Our blood is around 90% water and our lymphatic fluid (our waste disposal system) around 96% water. If we are even slightly dehydrated the blood and lymph fluid thickens, reducing delivery of oxygen and nutrients to the body and brain as the blood moves more slowly. The sludgier lymph fluid will also carry waste away from our organs more slowly, leading to higher levels of toxicity circulating in the brain for longer.

A great first step is to get into the habit of when you wake up always having a large glass of warm water – about body temperature, which you can judge by whether it feels neither hot not cold against your finger – with the juice of half a lemon or lime. A tiny pinch of sea or rock salt (not so much that the water tastes salty) is a great addition as it adds minerals, making the water more user-friendly for your body. This combo is highly hydrating, freshening up your system and helping eliminate toxins that have accumulated throughout the night. Use a straw to protect your tooth enamel from the citric acid. Then throughout the day aim to have sips of water alongside any tea or coffee and try to find some herbal teas so you're not so dependent on caffeine-based drinks, which can be dehydrating and overly stimulating. It's best not to drink large volumes of fluids while eating, as this can impair good digestion. Small sips are fine.

Many whole foods contain a lot of water, so you can eat your way to being better hydrated as well as drinking. Anything that absorbs water, like soaked chia and flax seeds, cooked beans and lentils, overnight-soaked oats or quinoa, will have lots of water held within the fibre. Fresh fruit and vegetables are water rich too. Think of a cucumber or a tomato, packed with what is called 'structured' water, held within the cells of the plant and very hydrating. By adding lemon or lime juice and salt to your morning water, you are creating a similar 'structured' water. Kombucha and water kefir fermented drinks are also 'structured' and have the added benefit of live microbes, making them a great option if you find plain water too boring.

Eating your brain happy

Eating for a happy brain is not about weighing foods, counting calories or measuring macros. It is about adding in more of what makes for a happy gut and reducing foods that can damage the gut. Rather than thinking that everything you currently do has to change, focus on how the foods and meals you already like to eat can be easily tweaked by including one or more of the types of food on the Eat Your Brain Happy list at every meal:

> **Eat Your Brain Happy**
>
> Include at every meal one or more of the following, combined with minimally processed proteins and healthy fats:
>
> - A broad range of whole plant foods
> - Bitter-tasting and richly coloured foods
> - Fermented foods

Remember the happy brain plate from the beginning of this chapter for what to aim for:

- ⅓ - ½ a variety of low starch (low sugar) plant-based foods + some fermented veggies
- ⅓ protein-rich foods
- ⅙ - ⅓ nutrient-rich starchy foods
- Topped off with some healthy fats and spices, toppings (or treats)

And to give you some ideas, here's a quick recap of my favourite happy brain superfoods. You can layer up and combine these ingredients in all sorts of ways. If a dish you're making or a recipe you're trying doesn't include one or more of these superhero foods, add a small amount and see how it tastes.

- **Eggs**
  A complete food that is unique in having every nutrient we need to make a brain cell. Egg yolks contain healthy fats and the white and yolk contain protein. Eggs also have a high level of choline, a B vitamin that is essential for making a brain chemical called acetylcholine, which supports brain cell communication, protects the liver and supports heart and muscle function.
- **Wild oily fish**
  Oily fish have a high protein content and, more critically, are high in omega 3 fatty acids, making them a must to include several times a week wherever possible. Choose sardines, mackerel, anchovies, wild salmon and herring – think SMASH. Tuna, swordfish and king mackerel are also sources of omega 3 but are not recommended on a regular basis due to toxins accumulated from living in contaminated waters. While smoked fish like smoked mackerel and smoked salmon will have lost much of their omega 3, eating canned oily fish appears to offer the same benefits as eating fresh fish. Opt

for whole fillets canned in spring water or olive oil rather than sunflower oil or brine.

- **Red meat, liver and bone broth**

  Red meat and liver have high levels of protein and lots of vitamins and minerals, especially B_{12}, zinc, iron and vitamin A, and omega 3 if grass fed. Minced beef, lamb, pork and venison are good choices, reasonably priced and very versatile. Add lots of vegetables, spices and herbs to make a simple, deeply nutritious dish. Cheaper cuts of meat are often more nutrient dense and higher in gut-mending collagen. These require long, slow cooking to break down the tough bits, but they are more nutritious than lean-muscle white meats like chicken breast. Put them in a slow cooker or low oven with some onions, carrots, garlic and rosemary, add a little stock or water and leave for several hours for a tender, brain-calming stew.

  Liver has high levels of iron, vitamin A and vitamin D. Adding small amounts of minced liver to minced beef (you can ask your butcher to add 5–10% liver) for a stew, burgers or meatballs is a great way to hide it if a slice of pan-fried liver is too unappealing. Good-quality pâté is also a great way to get some liver into the diet. A little goes a long way, though, so don't be tempted to have liver more than once a week and only consume in small amounts on rare occasions, once a month or so, if pregnant.

  Bone broth contains stacks of nutrients as well as some very specific amino acids that help fuel and seal the cells that line the gut and brain barriers, preventing them from becoming 'leaky'. A true bone broth will have been gently simmered for many hours, 12 hours minimum for small bones like chicken and at least 24 hours for bigger bones like beef and lamb. Drink the liquid hot or use for any recipes where stock is required, such as soups and stews. Many brands are now available to buy ready-made fresh or frozen, in powder or

jelly form. Get the best quality you can afford, as what the animals were fed is locked inside their bones.

- **Watercress and rocket (arugula)**
Dark leafy greens in general and watercress and rocket in particular have high levels of fibre and polyphenols. These leaves are packed with antioxidants to protect the cells from damage and inflammation, plus lutein and zeaxanthin, which are protective of eye health and brain health, and B vitamins, especially folate (also called B9), which is essential for many chemical processes throughout the body and brain. These are not just salad ingredients but can be added at the end of cooking to any dish where you would use spinach. They wilt down and may be more digestible if you find too much of these fibre-rich foods cause bloating.

- **Broccoli and other brassicas**
Broccoli is full of B vitamins, vitamin C, minerals, fibre, antioxidants, anti-inflammatories and sulphur, a compound critical to good detoxification and therefore a favourite of the liver and the gut. There are several different types of broccoli, from tender stem and broccolini, which are young and sweet and less likely to cause bloating, to purple sprouting, which is indeed purple and has very high levels of antioxidants. Romanesco, a cruciferous vegetable somewhere between broccoli and cauliflower, has geometric florets that look like fancy pyramids and is slightly sweeter than broccoli. Don't forget the other brassicas – cauliflower, cabbages, kale, bok choy and Brussel sprouts – which also have a high B vitamin content and a range of fibre.

- **Sprouted seeds and pulses**
I explained how to sprout beans and seeds earlier in the chapter, but broccoli sprouts deserve a special mention because they are very high in a compound called sulforaphane. This potent phytochemical is only activated once we chew it up and expose it to our gut microbes. Highly antioxidant and

incredibly anti-inflammatory, the small size of the compound allows it to pass through the blood–brain barrier, reduce neuroinflammation and protect against oxidative damage, both associated with depression and anxiety. It is very easy to sprout broccoli seeds at home and these peppery little plants are also readily available in many supermarkets. Simply soak 2 tablespoons of broccoli seeds in water overnight in a glass jar with a lid. Drain the water using a fine sieve or kitchen paper and then keep the jar away from direct light. Rinse the seeds once a day by swirling fresh water around the jar and then drain. Let them grow to about 2–3 cm, transfer to the fridge and use within a few days.

- **Pumpkin seeds**
  Pumpkin seeds contain good levels of zinc, essential for tissue healing, immune function regulation, hormone production and mental health. It is quick and easy to add them to salads, yogurt, snacks etc. to top up your zinc on a regular basis. Pumpkin seeds also contain good levels of gut-friendly fibre, protein and healthy fats, antioxidants and magnesium, which helps with mood, stress and sleep.
- **Chia and flax seeds**
  Chia seeds contain a high level of calcium, a good level of zinc and excellent amounts of the amino acid tryptophan, one of the main precursor nutrients to serotonin and melatonin production in the brain. They also have large amounts of omega 3 fatty acids, as well as a substance called caffeic acid, known to have anti-inflammatory benefits. You can add them to yogurt or muesli, or even use them as a topping for ice cream, but soaking first is highly advisable, as if not they will absorb fluid from your intestine, which can result in reduced transit time or even constipation and bowel irritation.

Flax seeds (aka linseeds) are also rich in omega 3 fatty acids and magnesium and are packed with fibre. They contain a wide range of phytochemicals called lignans, a type of polyphenol that are antioxidant, anti-inflammatory and hormone regulating. Grinding further increases the benefit, but do be cautious about buying pre-ground flax or flax meal. Due to the high content of omega 3 fats, it can easily turn rancid. Ideally grind your own or buy in small amounts, in opaque packaging, and keep in a cool, dry place. As with chia seeds, pre-soak and mix with yogurt, into smoothies or use in breakfast bowls. Do not heat.

- **Very dark chocolate and raw cacao nibs or powder**
  Chocolate can be a daily feature of happy brain eating if you are careful about your choices. Chocolate that has a high cocoa content will almost always have a low sugar content; milk chocolate has negligible levels of healthy compounds as well as more sugar. Cocoa contains lots of magnesium, polyphenols and flavonoids, which are thought to increase blood flow to the brain. It also contains tryptophan, the precursor to serotonin, plus anandamide, a brain chemical associated with feeling bliss and increasing oxytocin, the love and connection chemical. Packed with antioxidants, dark chocolate contains many compounds known to be protective against oxidative damage and various kinds of fibre. If you hate the bitter taste of dark chocolate, begin with a medium cocoa content, around 45–50% (it will clearly state this on the wrapper), and then nudge up to 60–70%. Before you know it you'll be actively enjoying a brain-healthy 85%+. Ideally have chocolate after meals and not too close to bedtime, as cocoa does contain some caffeine.
  Cacao is the bean that once roasted becomes cocoa. Due to the lack of processing, raw cacao, often sold as little chunks called nibs, has higher levels of nutrients and protective compounds, especially flavonoids. Its gritty bitterness can be unpleasant, but you can easily add cacao nibs to a breakfast bowl or muesli mix and you won't know they're there, or

use raw cacao powder in smoothies and recipes that require cocoa powder.

- **Green tea and matcha**
  Green tea is made from the same tea leaves as black tea but the processing is different, resulting in very high levels of antioxidant, anti-inflammatory and other protective compounds and lower caffeine. Specifically, a compound called epigallocatechin gallate (EGCG) is far higher in green tea than black tea and considerably higher in a specific type of green tea known as matcha, which is a vibrant green and is used in traditional Japanese tea ceremonies. As EGCG can pass across the blood–brain barrier it has direct effects on the brain, offering neuroprotective benefit and brain cell connectivity. Green tea has the added benefit of the amino acid L-theanine, which helps calm a ruminating brain and as such can counteract the buzz of caffeine, resulting in a focused and tranquil state. You can buy matcha green tea as a powder that can be added to smoothies or yogurt or made into tea. Many green teas have added herbs to make them more palatable. Try different brands to find one you really enjoy and aim to have a few cups a day, ideally before mid-afternoon just in case the caffeine affects your sleep.

- **Raw apple cider vinegar**
  Full of good microbes and digestive enzymes, raw apple cider vinegar can support digestion from top to bottom as well as having a generalised anti-inflammatory effect. A shot of 1 teaspoon to 1 tablespoon in a little water just before eating helps reduce the blood glucose response to starchy and sugary foods while also increasing stomach acid and enzyme secretions, improving protein digestion – especially useful if it's a late, heavy meal and/or carb rich. A good, live apple cider vinegar will be cloudy and contain sediment, and does not need to be chilled like other fermented foods.

- **Garlic and ginger (and spices in general)**
  These are two powerhouses for their anti-inflammatory and antioxidant effects. They not only add flavour to foods, they contain a complex range of phytochemicals, prebiotic fibre and polyphenols that offer cardiovascular protection while supporting the good gut microbes to thrive while helping to keep the bad bugs at bay.
- **Black (cumin) seed oil**
  The many health benefits of black seed oil were discussed earlier in the chapter. With so much to gain from it you may want to consider taking it as a supplement at a dose of 1–2 teaspoons several times a week. It is classed as a culinary oil, so you can include it in your range of good fats for salad dressings or smoothies – use the same criteria as for good olive oil, in that it should be cold pressed, organic, in a dark bottle and kept in a cool dark place.

CHAPTER SEVEN
Unhappy Brain Foods and How to Avoid Them

Chapter Six described how to nourish ourselves day to day for a happy brain, but it's also helpful to know what not to eat and drink. This chapter takes a look at the unhappy brain foods that could be getting in the way of your mental health, and offers strategies for minimising and avoiding them.

Highly processed foods

Ultra-processed foods have been much discussed in the media and scientific world recently. In this book I use the more understandable term highly processed foods, but they mean the same. Much of the food we consume undergoes some form of processing, including pasteurising, canning or baking, but the difference with highly processed foods is that they contain a long list of ingredients, many of which are almost unrecognisable as food and would not be on the shelf in your kitchen, including artificial sweeteners, emulsifiers and flavourings. Many of these ingredients are known to be toxic to the gut microbes and irritating to the gut lining, as well as affecting brain chemistry, and the effects of a large number of them in varying combinations cannot be known.

Examples of highly processed foods range from fizzy drinks to ice cream, ready meals to breakfast cereals, crisps to confectionery. They can be highly addictive; in fact some are specifically engineered to be that way. They tend to contain large amounts of some of the other foods on the unhappy brain foods list, including sugar and artificial sweeteners, refined grains and refined oils. A good rule of thumb is to avoid foods with more than five ingredients, and especially those that include things you don't recognise or can't pronounce.

Refined grains

No human being requires any grains to be healthy, but we do tend to love the stodgy foods made from grains such as bread, pasta, sushi, porridge and risotto. Grains like wheat, rice, oats or corn in any form can be disruptive to the gut and brain, as grains in general are aggressive on blood glucose, are low in nutrients and can be aggravating to a sensitive gut. If a grain is refined the fibre and nutrients have been removed. The whole, 'brown' versions of rice and wheat are commonly considered healthier, but this is not necessarily the case. The inclusion of the outer husk allows a grain to be termed whole even if it's then been pulverised into flour, flakes, puffed or pre-cooked. The impact on blood sugar is much greater the more processed the grain, whether whole or refined. A food doesn't have to taste sweet to become sugar in your system – your saliva turns starches like grains into the equivalent of sugar in your mouth. You can test this out: if you allow a bite of a rice cake to dissolve in your mouth you will rapidly taste sugar; if you chew a mouthful of bread for long enough it will taste sweet.

Look for whole, un- or minimally processed grains and maybe consider having a total break from all grains for a few weeks to see how you feel. Some people find avoiding grains entirely to be a significant benefit to the body and brain. It's fine to have them now and again, but understand that they are not providing good fuel and may be affecting your mood and energy.

Wheat is the most popular grain in the UK and is worth addressing in a section of its own.

Wheat and gluten

Wheat provides us with many of our comfort foods: bread, pasta, cakes, biscuits, pastries, breakfast cereals, crispy coatings and traditional puddings. Most people will be fine with eating some wheat, some of the time. However, many people feel a lot, lot better if they stay off it completely.

There is a difference between being wheat free and being gluten free. Gluten is a protein found in wheat, rye and barley, which increases shelf-life and improves the texture of bread and other wheat-based products. However, humans don't make an enzyme to break this protein down, rendering it a gut irritant. Rye and barley are not consumed to the same extent as wheat and despite them containing a little gluten, many people feel fine when they eat them now and again. Wheat, however, is often eaten multiple times a day in various forms and has a far higher gluten content. It also contains high levels of glyphosate, a chemical that is sprayed on wheat and other crops as a pesticide and to dry crops before storage. Both gluten and glyphosate consumed on a regular basis can he highly problematic, even for those who have no actual food sensitivity or allergic response to gluten or wheat.

After consuming wheat the symptoms most commonly experienced are bloating and abdominal pain, a severe energy crash, brain fog and/or confused thinking and overwhelm, and food or sugar cravings. These can be due to numerous factors:

- Wheat, even whole wheat, causing high spikes in blood glucose followed by energy-sapping and brain-numbing crashes.
- Gluten is known to cause, or worsen, gut permeability (leaky gut; see Chapter Three), where the cells that line the gut wall open up, allowing food particles and pathogens to pass into the bloodstream. This can trigger a lot of inflammation around the body and brain.
- Gluten is digested into opioid-like products (gluteomorphins), causing wheat-based foods to be literally very addictive, resulting in cravings and over-eating.
- Glyphosate is an antibiotic and is therefore harmful to the

beneficial gut microbes. It is also very aggressive on the gut lining, increasing gut permeability alongside gluten.

If you eat a lot of wheat, try giving up both wheat and gluten completely for a few weeks to allow for a brain reset. The difference in your energy can be felt within a week or so of being entirely gluten free. Giving up gluten often helps or resolves many digestive issues too and facilitates fat loss. Then after a few weeks try a little rye bread and see how you feel. If you have no mental or physical effects within 24 hours of eating the rye, try some wheat. Have a meal with a wheat-based food and notice how you feel over the following 24 hours. You might have no issues, suggesting you are fine with wheat and gluten. However, if the wheat causes you issues, you know it's the wheat rather than gluten that's the problem because you were fine with the rye.

Don't be tempted to replace all your beloved wheat-based foods with gluten-free look-a-likes, as they are often highly processed (look at the ingredients list: the fewer the better). Bean- and lentil-based pastas are a great alternative, seed-based breads are a much better choice and consider making some simple home-baked goodies that are low in sugar and wheat free. There are endless resources online for wheat- and gluten-free ideas – see the resources list at the back of this book.

Refined cooking oils

Refined cooking oils such as rapeseed (canola) oil, sunflower oil, corn oil, grapeseed oil, vegetable oil and soybean oil are everywhere. Consuming the seeds in their natural form – for instance eating whole sunflower seeds – is not the issue, it's the way the oil is extracted from the seeds. Rather than the traditional cold pressing used to obtain such products as extra virgin olive oil, refined cooking oils are produced using heat and solvents, then degummed, deodorised, bleached and filtered. This renders once-healthy oils highly damaged and damaging to humans.

Excess use of these oils is associated with inflammation and an increase in oxidative stress, a 'rusting' of our insides. Don't use them in your own kitchen, and read labels carefully to avoid products that contain them.

Alcohol

A comforting crutch for many people, alcohol is not a friend to the happy brain. It is well documented to be a depressant due to its dysregulating effect on numerous 'feel-good' brain chemicals. It disrupts our gut microbes, places a burden on the liver, which then affects our fat burning and blood glucose systems, causes inflammation in the brain and depletes nutrients. Combine this with the likelihood that your resolve to eat and live well will be weakened under the influence of alcohol, and it really is something you may want to greatly limit or avoid.

Abstinence is not absolutely necessary, although it is hard to make a convincing argument that any amount of alcohol serves a useful purpose other than the fleeting pleasure it can bring. As a sedative and relaxant, alcohol can help ease symptoms of anxiety and the intoxication it provides can serve to temporarily distract from the hardships we face. Having some alcohol on an occasional basis is probably not causing long-term harm, but alcohol on a regular basis – nightly or most nights of the week – could be.

Many people are staggered how much better they feel once they take the leap, break the habit and enjoy the benefits of better sleep, better metabolic health, lower body fat, better liver function and so much more. If you do choose to consume alcohol:

- Aim for at least four nights off a week
- Only drink once you have some food in your system
- Match the volume of alcohol with at least as much water
- Be very present when drinking, so that you sip, enjoy and appreciate the moment

Sugar

Sugar is an entirely unnecessary component of our diet. We have no need whatsoever for it. Many people love sweet foods and believe their 'sweet tooth' is an irrepressible trait that can never be overcome – not so. We do all have a primal drive to love and pursue sweetness, especially sweet, fatty foods, because that's what breast milk consists of. This sweet, cholesterol-rich, growth-promoting bounty is the perfect blend of fats and sugars to stimulate the addictive region of the brain, the nucleus accumbens, ensuring newborns love the taste of their mother's milk and keep going back for more. A well-fed baby is a happy and healthy baby. However, mother nature does not combine sugars and fats in any other way, rendering that sugar–fat-addicted part of the brain redundant once the baby is weaned. It's only with the influx of modern processed foods that the sugar–fat hit, devoid of anything nutritious yet highly available, as often as we choose, is driving the desire to eat these foods far beyond what we need.

If we eat sugar and sweet-tasting foods on a regular basis, we increase that drive for sugar. The brain becomes hardwired to want it, seek it out and devour it. A sugar hit can provide a boost of feel-good brain chemicals as well as a surge of physical energy when we're feeling tired. It makes perfect sense why we love it and want it. That does not, however, mean it's good for our mental or physical health.

It is entirely possible to switch your 'sweet tooth' off and get to a place where you genuinely, without effort or willpower, actively choose not to have regular hits of sweetness. Once you break the cycle of sugar addiction your taste buds, brain receptors and gut microbes all adjust accordingly, freeing you from the compulsive behaviours and subsequent emotional, mental and physical rollercoasters of overly consuming sugar.

In all its many forms, from white table sugar to the seemingly not so bad honey or agave syrup, it is best to limit and avoid sugar wherever possible. If you look at the back of a packet of food and sugar is anywhere within the first five ingredients, avoid it. It's also worth noting that sugar comes in many guises, often with -ose at the end. Fructose, sucrose and glucose syrup are common, but also look out for dextrose, maltose, maltodextrin, invert sugar syrup, malt syrup, any syrup or treacle. There are currently over 100 names for sugar in food labelling, so don't just look for 'sugar' in the ingredients list.

Many books have been written on the subject of sugar and films have even been made about its addictive qualities and ability to wreck our metabolism. That Sugar Film (2015) is a fun watch, great for children and still relevant as it makes very clear the stark reality of how the food industry can manipulate our tastebuds and emotional regulation with its insidious marketing and highly palatable sugary goods.

> **Sugar intake**
>
> *The World Health Organisation (WHO) recommends that people of all ages reduce their sugar intake to less than 10% of daily calories, which translates roughly to 50 g per day for adults eating 2000 calories a day. That is equivalent to 10 teaspoons of sugar. WHO does state that a further reduction to 5% or 5 teaspoons per day would be preferable. This is not necessarily added teaspoons of sugar in your coffee and tea. It's the total added sugar in your foods like breakfast cereals, yogurts, jam, honey, biscuits, cakes, pasta and curry sauces, salad cream and so much more.*

How much sugar are you really eating?

Five teaspoons is certainly a great goal. If you are interested in assessing how much you are consuming on top of any sugar you're adding to your food and drinks, look at the nutrition data label of any packet foods you buy. You will see listed there total carbohydrates and added sugars. To understand how much sugar is in that food, make sure you check the serving size: it's rare that a serving size is what people actually eat, it's often half that amount. If a food has 10 g of added sugar per serving, that's equivalent to 2 teaspoons of sugar (1 teaspoon = 5 g). You'll be amazed at how quickly those teaspoons of sugar add up, especially if you get really good at checking all your packaged foods. There's added sugar in some brands of crisps, corn chips, oven fries, pickles and even so-called savoury dips, soups, breads and crackers. Ketchups, dressings and many other 'non-sweet' foods often have sugars added too.

GEEK BOX

Net carbs vs sugar carbs

The amount of added sugar in a food is not the same as the total amount of sugar (glucose) that goes into the bloodstream from that food. Remember, it's not just sugar that turns into blood sugar, the glucose in starches does too. This is an important distinction because a food could have 'no added sugar' but lots of corn starch or rice flour. These ingredients rapidly turn to sugar in your body but are not included in the total sugar amount. This is what we call net carbs, the amounts of carbohydrates that turn into sugar in your blood.

To work out the glucose hit to your bloodstream as opposed to the sugar added to the food, you need to work out the net carbohydrate level. This is calculated by subtracting any fibre grams that are listed from the total carbohydrates per serving. Fibre grams can be deducted because they are part of the total carbohydrate count but aren't absorbed, so they don't add to the sugar burden in the blood. Once you have the net carbohydrates per portion (not the same as per packet), divide by 5 to get the equivalent teaspoons because 5 g = 1 teaspoon. More than 1 teaspoon of sugar in the blood and your body is having to manage this excess sugar, which could be irritating your brain.

For instance, the following nutritional data is taken from a box of 'low-sugar' granola:

Typical Values	Per 100 g	Per 40 g (a suggested serving)
Energy	1727 kj/411 kcal	691 kj/164 kcal
Carbohydrate	62 g	25 g
Of which sugars	3.1 g	1.2 g
Fibre	13 g	5.0 g

The sugars per serving are very low, only 1.2 g. However, the net carbs are 20 g: total carbs (25) minus fibre (5) = 20. Divide by 5 and you have the equivalent of 4 teaspoons of sugar hitting the bloodstream. In this example, the net carbs are coming from refined oats and maple syrup – that's still sugar.

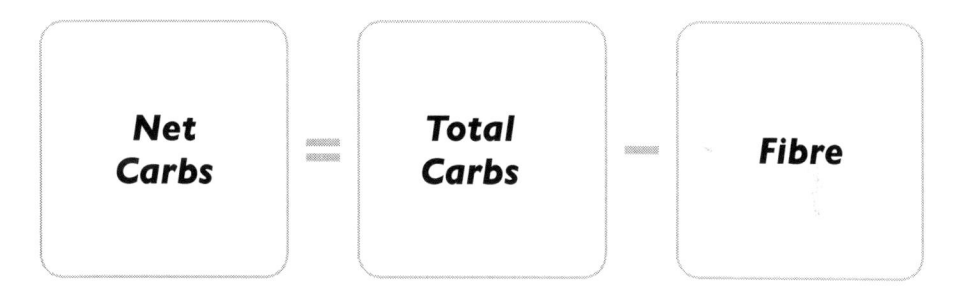

Net Carbs = **Total Carbs** − **Fibre**

Here are just a few reasons why you might benefit from quitting or cutting down on sugar:

- Sugar provides nothing of nutritional use and depletes the body of nutrients in the process of being digested. Therefore, we are in a nutrient deficit after eating sugar.
- Sugar provides a very quick burst of energy as it turns into blood glucose (sugar in the blood) extremely quickly. While this can provide a physical and mental high, it will be rapidly followed by a mighty crash.

- Sugar feeds undesirable, pathogenic microbes in the gut, which then begin to crowd out the good 'happy' microbes. This can lead to an undesirable state of gut bug imbalance known as dysbiosis, a well-known causal factor of depression and anxiety.
- Sugar causes inflammation throughout the body. Inflammation is associated with all chronic diseases including cancer and with depression.
- Sugar can impair the immune system, including the immune system of the brain, our glial cells, which can lead to brain inflammation associated with mental health disorders.
- Sugar is literally chemically addictive – the more you have the more you will want.
- Excess sugar consumption over prolonged periods can cause diabetes. Alzheimer's is now being termed diabetes of the brain or type 3 diabetes, and there is a lot of research looking into this mechanism in anxiety and depression.
- High sugar levels in the brain can create blockages across our synapses, the gap between our neurons (brain cells) where our brain chemicals are exchanged.
- High sugar intake can cause neurons to misfire, sending wonky signals that the brain must work hard to correct.
- High levels of blood glucose damage the blood vessels and cells. This is why the body will try to clear the sugar we've eaten from our blood as quickly as possible, but it often overcompensates. The blood sugar low that follows causes brain and body fatigue, cravings for more sugar and low and anxious mood.

If you think you are a sugar addict or simply cannot imagine life without sweet foods because sugar is a critical provider of pleasure and energy for you, understand that it is entirely possible to get to a point where avoiding sugar is no longer a challenge. I appreciate this can be very hard to believe for life-long sugar lovers, but I know from helping very many sugar-dependent people how relatively quickly this can be resolved and how incredibly liberating it is too. As with any addictive substance, if you can avoid it, you can retrain your brain not to crave it. But unlike alcohol and drugs, sugar can be much harder to avoid.

Start with the refined, added sugar found in sweet foods and many packaged savoury foods. Breakfast cereals are notorious for being loaded with multiple forms of sugar. Don't forget about your drinks: sodas, tonics and energy drinks are often sugar bombs. If there are zero sugars in a food or drink, check the ingredients list for artificial sweeteners, as you want to be avoiding these too.

Artificial sweeteners

Despite being calorie free, artificial sweeteners are not by any means healthy. Not only are they associated with several potential health issues for the heart and the gut, anything that tastes sweet stimulates the sweet taste buds on the tongue, which perpetuates a drive for sugar and sweet-tasting foods. If you get cravings for something sweet, artificially sweetened drinks and foods can make these worse and keep your brain locked into the sugar pleasure drive. So read labels carefully and consume these products moderately, if at all.

> **GEEK BOX**
>
> **Artificial sweeteners**
>
> *Artificial sweeteners were first touted as a health food as they provided sweet-tasting foods for diabetics without causing blood sugar issues. Calorie free and cheap, these sweet chemical compounds became very popular in the 1960s. As research findings resulted in one type of artificial sweetener being banned for various health concerns, including cancer, another was developed. A report in the British Medical Journal in 2022 revealed the results of a study conducted in France from 2009 to 2021 showing a significant increase in cardiovascular disease in relation to*

artificial sweetener consumption. [55] *Another French study of over 66,000 women found that those who regularly consumed artificially sweetened drinks doubled their risk of type 2 diabetes* [56] *– ironic, but not so hard to understand when you think of the body's internal communication system. If our tastebuds taste something super-sweet, the message to the brain is that we are consuming sugar – we have no taste buds for chemical-based sweeteners. The brain then actions the body to respond as if we were having sugar. Over time this can result in weight gain and insulin resistance, two big risk factors for type 2 diabetes. A more recent, very troubling study from Israel, where a lot of research is conducted on the gut microbiome, found that the gut microbes' metabolism of artificial sweeteners produces a toxic by-product that kills off our good gut bugs.* [57]

Artificial sweetener brands

In the UK:
Canderel – contains aspartame

Splenda – contains sucralose
Sweetex – contains saccharin

In the USA:
Nutrasweet & Equal
– contains aspartame
Splenda – contains sucralose
Sweet'N Low, Sweet Twin /
Sugar Twin – contain saccharin

When temptation strikes

If you find you are longing for foods that are on the unhappy brain foods list that you think of as delicious, mood enhancing, energy giving or simply pleasurable and a treat, try to make sense of why they are not supportive of your long-term well-being. Make it a positive choice not to have those foods based on you making a decision for your own benefit, rather than seeing it as something you have to deny yourself because you're being told to by someone else.

When you are eating these foods, the cycle of effects looks like this:

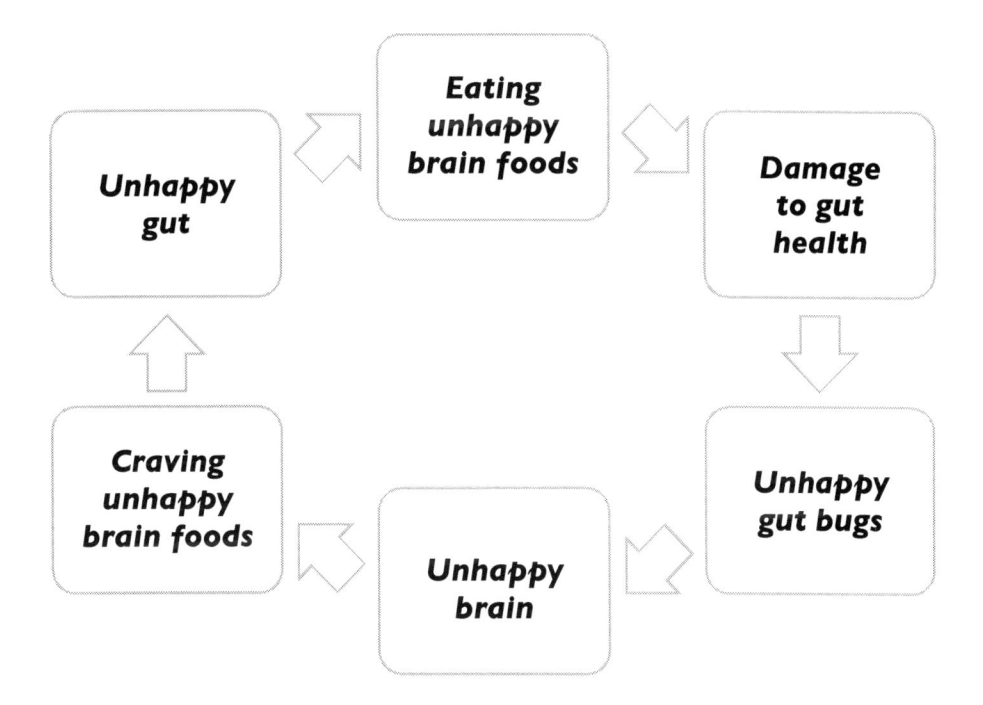

```
        ┌─────────────┐
        │   Eating    │
        │  unhappy    │
        │ brain foods │
        └─────────────┘
       ↗               ↘
┌──────────┐         ┌──────────┐
│ Unhappy  │         │  Damage  │
│   gut    │         │  to gut  │
│          │         │  health  │
└──────────┘         └──────────┘
     ↑                     ↓
┌──────────┐         ┌──────────┐
│ Craving  │         │ Unhappy  │
│ unhappy  │         │ gut bugs │
│brain foods│        │          │
└──────────┘         └──────────┘
       ↖               ↙
        ┌─────────────┐
        │   Unhappy   │
        │    brain    │
        └─────────────┘
```

Breaking this cycle is paramount. The more you don't have these foods, the easier it gets not to have them, honestly. The healthier your gut bugs, the more balanced your brain chemistry, the less of a drive you feel for quick-fix, so-called treat foods – because your body and brain are managing your happy balance better. It's like a skill that, once learnt, you don't have to work hard at.

I believe everyone can get to the point where food choices and meal plans become entirely instinctive because our lived experience confirms what we need to eat to keep us on track for a happy brain. But you may feel like you are so far off right now that it's overwhelming even to think about where to start. Go back to the starting point of greatly reducing sugar, refined grains and processed foods. Just begin, one meal at a time, to swap out ingredients and balance your meals better. Then get going on the 3Fs: start with Fibre, then think about Fermented foods, and at some point you'll be ready to take on Fasting too.

Think about how hard you had to concentrate when you first learnt to drive, or knit or ride a bike, compared to how automatic these things become once you're well practised. The most difficult time is now, as you are trying to integrate this new information into your life and working out what it means for you day to day. Soon it will become second nature.

Enjoy your food

There are some small changes to *how* you eat that will help you become more tuned in to what to eat and when, so you focus on what you *can* eat rather than what you're trying to avoid. They fall into two categories: what do to more of and what to do less of when eating.

What to do more of when eating...

Ask yourself if you're hungry

We all eat for reasons other than hunger: boredom, an energy crash, feeling sad, feeling down, feeling lost, unloved, dissatisfied with life or simply the time of day. Eating can provide momentary pleasure and distraction from feelings and thoughts that are uncomfortable. Some foods can literally change our brain chemistry to produce more pleasure and happiness hormones. In fact, food manufacturers work hard to make foods that hit the 'bliss point' – a combination of factors that create a moreish high. These have the classic combination of sugars and fats, often coupled with a crunch. Whether it's ice cream, biscuits, crisps, corn chips, milk chocolate or pizza, these all trigger the brain to want more.

Ask yourself why you are longing for these foods. If it's because you really are hungry, try to find an alternative food source. Salty, bitter, savoury foods coupled with protein are a great way to break a sugar craving. If you realise you're not actually hungry but are looking for a hit of pleasure, find a healthy distraction that feels good but doesn't involve food, such as listening to some of your favourite music or contacting a friend.

Take a moment

Even before you begin eating, the biofeedback between your brain and your digestive system can be actioned through smelling, looking at and anticipating what you are about to eat, so pause and focus on your food before you take your first mouthful. Saliva floods into the mouth in preparation for eating. But you don't produce saliva when you're in fight-or-flight mode. In fact, your mouth can become noticeably dry when high levels of stress kick in – your lips stick to your teeth, making it hard to talk properly, never mind eat properly.

The 'gear' you need to be in when eating and digesting is entirely opposite to the gear of doing, rushing, driving, reading, watching TV, answering emails, chatting on the phone. You need to be present, engaged and focused on the food you are about to eat to allow the rest-and-digest 'parasympathetic' arm of the nervous system, governed by the vagus nerve, to begin to action the process of digestion. That entails turning off your fight-or-flight, 'sympathetic' nervous system signals by creating a moment of calm before tucking in. Crucially, with this also comes a heightened sense of taste and pleasure, hence a greater appreciation of our food.

So, turn off your devices, put away your work, settle yourself comfortably with your food on a table in front of you (not on your lap ideally) and take a few deep breaths in through your nose and out through your mouth. And relax. Notice your food, smell your food, have a moment of gratitude for your food before you begin to eat.

Chew

This may not be the most exciting of recommendations, but it's so, so important. Even the healthiest diet can be problematic if the food that you swallow isn't chewed enough. It's not just the mechanics of your teeth grinding down your food that make chewing so instrumental in healthy digestion, it is also the food mixing with saliva, which helps break it down and eases its passage down the throat to the stomach. Chewing also gives your taste buds a chance to acknowledge what you're eating, which sends signals to the brain, which then actions the stomach to make appropriate levels of stomach acid and protein-digesting enzymes to further digest the food.

Pause between mouthfuls

Again, not a super-sexy suggestion but very effective. Take time to pause between mouthfuls – a great tip is to put your cutlery down between each bite. This gives your stomach time to send signals to your brain that you've had enough, via a response to being stretched. If you eat quickly, you can easily over-stuff your stomach before you get the feeling of fullness. Over time you can get used to feeling very full and you then expect to reach this level of fullness every time you eat.

The stomach is a flexible and stretchy bag and if you eat slowly it's surprising how quickly you can reset your fullness factor by stimulating a stronger stretch response to kick in more rapidly. If you are a bolter (many people are), then set yourself the goal of being the last to finish when eating in company.

What to do less of when eating

- Don't eat on the move, when distracted, in the car
- Don't look at a TV, computer or phone screen
- Don't grab and go – put your food on a plate
- Don't graze throughout the day – make proper meals
- Don't drink a large volume of water during or just after eating
- Don't fill your fork for the next mouthful until your mouth is empty
- Don't continue to eat once you're feeling full
- Don't feel you need to empty your plate

A conscious treat

For some people it's important to know that they can have some of their 'treat' unhappy brain foods now and again – and I say an absolute yes to that. Keep in mind that it's your choice if and when you have some of your favourite foods that you know might not be the best for your mental well-being. If you do make this choice now and again, do it consciously, with awareness, and most of all enjoy it. And bear in mind that often people get tempted to have one of their past treat foods, only to find not only is it no longer pleasurable to eat, but the after-effects of how it makes them feel affirm that there's no place for this food in their diet any longer.

Here are some things you can do to mitigate any harmful effects if you do indulge in a treat:

- Eat the very best version of your treat food possible. Plan ahead so you have what you really want and don't compromise – make it count and check in with yourself to see if you actually enjoy it as much as you think.
- Eat your chosen 'unhappy' food after eating something really gut supportive.
- Eat really slowly and with focus so you don't miss the experience, otherwise you'll end up wanting more.
- Take a suitable portion, put it on a plate or in a bowl, and then walk away or put the rest away so you're not continually tempted.
- Sit down to eat. Eating on the move, in a car, standing up or from the packet makes it so much easier to eat more than you intended because you're not engaging with the experience.
- Make sure you are well hydrated, which helps with satisfaction signals.
- Try to stay active for 15–20 minutes after eating.

Plan your indulgences: make them count. If you eat a 'treat', make it a conscious choice. Get the best quality you can, notice it and savour it.

One of the most important aspects of your happy brain action plan is to view it as a positive, lasting change rather than something you resent having to do. It feels great to feel great, so pause before you decide to eat something that might throw you off kilter.

CHAPTER EIGHT
Strategic Supplementation

A supplement can rarely achieve major and lasting change without the foundations of a healthy diet and lifestyle being in place (we'll come to lifestyle in Chapter Nine). Think about supplements as an additional bonus to an already healthy diet – to top it up or fill in any gaps. It's an unfortunate reality that much of our food, even whole or minimally processed food, is not nearly as nutrient rich as it used to be, partly due to chronic depletion of nutrients in the soil. Add to that the effects of stress on our ability to digest and absorb the nutrients that are present in our foods, as well as certain genetic variations that increase the need for specific nutrients, and supplements are increasingly necessary to meet our daily requirements for optimal levels of nourishment. Careful, strategic supplementation can be a really helpful additional part of your happy brain action plan.

The recommended daily allowance or RDA, the amount of individual nutrients the government advises we should consume on a daily basis, is merely the amount needed not to get a disease associated with a deficiency, such as rickets caused by inadequate vitamin D or beriberi caused by low levels of vitamin B_1. This is nowhere near the amount we need for the body and brain to function and thrive at an optimal level. And again, what is optimal is individual and fluctuates throughout our life, so the main point is, it's complicated!

In this chapter I outline a basic protocol for a happy brain that almost everyone will benefit from, as it addresses the most consistently deficient nutrients in the modern diet. I then provide a brief explanation of some more specialist supplements that are associated with direct and indirect support of better mood, gut and brain function. It is difficult to give more individualised advice, so you may want to pursue professional help, which may require some blood tests, to determine any specific supplements you need. But first, a little background information.

Do supplements really work?

Studies conducted over the last few years at the University of Canterbury's Mental Health and Nutrition Research Lab in New Zealand, led by Julia Rucklidge, a professor of clinical psychiatry, have seen very good results in depressed volunteers using a high-quality multivitamin and mineral to supplement the diet. Ensuring optimal levels of vitamins D, A and E, the B vitamins and minerals such as zinc, selenium and iron proved highly effective at improving clinical markers of depression and anxiety. [58] Increasing vitamin D levels through supplementation was also shown to greatly improve recovery from traumatic events. Another team led by Professor Felice Jacka (who we met in the Introduction) studied the use of vitamin D, omega 3 and polyphenol-rich supplements for mental wellness. Measurable improvements were seen in the gut microbiome, which then presented as improved mood and behaviour. [59]

But while the benefits have been shown, there are hundreds of individual nutrients and blends being sold as 'brain healthy' or nootropic. There is little regulation in this area and a lot of hype, making it a bit of a lottery to choose what to take. Knowledge tends to confer better compliance, so this chapter is a guide to help you make better-informed choices.

It is always advisable to get some advice from a qualified and registered nutritional therapist and to check with your prescribing doctor if you are taking medication to ensure there are no contraindications. These are rare with food-based supplements, but not impossible.

The basic happy brain supplement protocol

- Multivitamin and mineral
- Methylated B complex
- Vitamin D_3 + K_2
- Omega 3 fish oil
- Magnesium

Multivitamin and mineral

Taking a good daily multivitamin and mineral supplement all of the time is a great idea to ensure you're covering any nutrient gaps in your diet. Too much of any one individual nutrient for too long and not enough of another can lead to problems over the long term, so a multi is generally a safe start.

In theory a multivitamin and mineral supplement will contain a percentage of all the essential vitamins and minerals we rely on from food as we cannot make them within the body, plus additional ingredients depending on the brand. That's a lot of ingredients to get into a very small pill or capsule, which tends to result in not very much of anything in each one. We do only need tiny amounts of some nutrients, the trace elements, whereas other nutrients, such as magnesium that is big and bulky, we need in much larger amounts.

The percentage of the RDA included per pill or per dose (often more than one pill) will be stated on the label. There is huge variability in how much of each nutrient there will be and critically in what form. This is important to consider as some forms are absorbed far better than others. Naturally sourced, as opposed to synthetically created, nutrients are more readily taken up by the body so much less is required per dose. However, it is unlikely you will ever see 'from synthetic sources' written on a label, as manufacturers of a cheaper option don't want to advertise that they use 'non-natural' ingredients.

So what do you need to look for?

- Food-based/wholefood/liposomal/bio-available or some version of these terms indicates a natural source as opposed to synthetic.
- If this is not clear, there's a clue to the quality of a product in the type of B vitamins listed on the back. If the product you are looking at has the more bio-available forms of B vitamins, then it's more likely to be a higher-quality product overall (see the next section on methylated B complex supplements for details on this).
- The ingredients list should also contain the trace minerals: chromium, selenium, copper, zinc, molybdenum, iodine and iron.
- Also check for vitamin D_3 – not D_2, which is less useful – and for vitamin K_2, which is important but is relatively expensive, so is often missing from cheaper products.
- A multivitamin and mineral in capsule or powder form is preferred to a pressed tablet.

Zinc

Many chronic mental health conditions improve with zinc supplementation and zinc also appears to improve the efficacy of anti-depressant drugs for those who do not otherwise experience benefit from them.[60] Zinc appears to be involved in numerous pathways that regulate neurotransmitter levels as well as new brain cell growth and is a protective antioxidant. Many people are zinc deficient, not just from a low intake of zinc-rich foods but also because it can be quite hard to absorb.

Iron

Research has found that *'Low iron has been clearly linked to depression well before levels are low enough to cause anaemia'*.[61] While supplementation might be advisable, there are many considerations to bear in mind:

- Some multis contain very small amounts of iron, less than 4 mg per serving (not per tablet), which is fine for most people as it is similar to levels naturally found in a balanced diet.
- Men and postmenopausal women tend not to need much if any extra iron, as too much is toxic and inflammatory.
- A small percentage of people have exceptionally high iron levels, usually genetically driven, and they should always take an iron-free multi.
- Those on a plant-based diet are far more likely to require additional iron than those who eat meat, although low stomach acid, commonly caused by chronic stress and antacid medications, can greatly inhibit iron absorption whatever the diet.

So some people will need iron supplementation in addition to what is contained in a multivitamin and mineral, but this should be taken separately so that the amount can be controlled.

Methylated B vitamins

Many mental health problems improve with higher B vitamin supplementation, beyond that found in even a very good multivitamin, making a vitamin B complex worth considering. This is simply all of the eight B vitamins in one capsule at much higher levels that those in a standard multi. As the B vitamins are water soluble, any excess the body can't use will be peed out. One's urine can turn quite a lurid yellow due to the body excreting vitamin B_2, but this is nothing to worry about.

To assess whether you benefit from this additional complex, see how you feel after 3–4 weeks of taking extra Bs. If there is no tangible change for the better, a multi along with a good diet may be sufficient.

The three big players for a happy brain are vitamins B6 (pantothenic acid), B9 (folate) and B12 (cobalamin). Like with a multi, it's not only about how much is present but in what form. A good form generally means you need less to do the job, so it's a false economy to pay less for a supplement only to discover you are getting little or no benefit because your body doesn't recognise the 'fake form' of what you should ideally be obtaining from your food. For a good B complex look at the ingredients list for these terms:

- Vitamin B6: pyridoxil-5-phosphate – often written as P-5-P or PLP – rather than pyridoxine hydrochloride.
- Vitamin B9: methylfolate or 5-methyltetrahydrofolic acid, not just folic acid.
- Vitamin B12: methylcobalamin or adenosylcobalamin rather than cyanocobalamin.

The family of eight B vitamins is involved in the conversion of food into energy, immune regulation, inflammatory responses, metabolic function and much more. They all have specific roles with many crossover functions. They are all essential and are found in many plant and animal foods, with the exception of vitamin B12, for which there are very few non-animal sources.

The importance of getting adequate and correct sources of these B vitamins daily cannot be understated.

A study from the University of Reading [62] showed that high doses of vitamin B6 reduced feelings of anxiety and depression in young people. David Field, the lead author, explained that vitamin B6 helps the chemical balance in the brain to produce more GABA, which calms brain activity. Crucially, despite many foods containing vitamin B6, such as tuna, chickpeas and many fruits and vegetables, the calming effects seen in this study came from very high levels that could not be achieved with food alone. The stimulation and excitation we are putting our brains through these days, with all the artificial light, screen time, stress load and foods becoming less nutrient dense, mean we have a far greater demand for the calming effects of vitamin B_6 than we did decades ago. Vitamin B_6 is also a co-factor in the production of serotonin, dopamine and other neurochemicals that affect our mood and brain energy.

> ***Vitamin B_6 is a precursor to serotonin, dopamine and GABA. Without enough B_6 our brains cannot make sufficient neurotransmitters to manage our mood and brain health.***

Vitamin B_9 (folate) has been well researched [63, 64] for its role in anxiety and depression. Low folate levels are linked to a poor response to antidepressants; conversely, there is a greater response to these medications when levels are high. Populations in areas of the world where diets are naturally high in these B vitamins consistently report a low prevalence of mood disorders.

> ***Good levels of vitamin B_9 (folate) improve patient response to antidepressant medication.***

Those on plant-based diets are very vulnerable to vitamin B_{12} deficiency because of the lack of non-animal sources, although it is becoming increasingly common across many populations even when animal products are consumed. This could be due to suppressed stomach acid levels (because of stress) reducing the absorption of vitamin B_{12}. Increasing vitamin B_{12} can significantly improve many neurological issues like nerve pain and tinnitus, as well as easing mental health symptoms. Higher levels of vitamin B_{12} are also associated with better treatment outcomes in physical medicine.

The B vitamins in general, and the 'big 3' in particular, are critical for the process of methylation, which allows millions of chemical transactions to take place where one brain chemical or hormone converts to another. Folate (vitamin B9) is needed in good and constant amounts to fuel this continuous chemical dance. However, folate can't do its job without its partners, vitamins B$_6$ and B$_{12}$. They are all integral to this life-saving process. Key examples of methylation include the conversion of tryptophan, an essential amino acid in food, to serotonin, the 'happy' brain chemical. Serotonin then converts to melatonin (which affects sleep) and glutamate converts to GABA (which calms the brain) through further methylation.

GEEK BOX

Methylation and folic acid

Methylation is a huge part of our metabolic system, allowing food to become energy through a complex process of conversion pathways. Methylation is also essential for managing our inflammatory responses, protection of our DNA, cardiovascular health, the ageing process, thyroid hormone activation and production of neurotransmitters – the brain chemicals we need for a happy brain.

Methylation also enables the conversion of folic acid (the synthetic form of vitamin B9 found in many supplements and fortified foods) to its active form, folate. However, there is a common genetic variant that affects how well someone methylates. Estimates vary from 45% to 80% of populations carrying one or two versions of the gene that slows or inhibits good methylation. What this means in practice is that those with this variant need higher amounts of the ready-to-go form of folate that is already methylated, methylfolate.

If you are a poor methylator, a great diet and a healthy gut can still leave you lacking in folate, which then affects the levels of many other happy brain nutrients. As vitamins B$_{12}$ and B$_6$ are critical co-factors in this complex and crucial system, ensuring you meet your needs with a good-quality supplement is an easy and essential first step to a happy brain.

> *Getting your homocysteine levels checked would help you see whether you methylate well: high homocysteine indicates poor methylation and a greater need for methylated B vitamins.*

Vitamin B_1, also known as thiamine, is in many different animal and plant-based foods but it's still possible to be deficient, especially if your digestion is not functioning well. The whole nervous system and many areas of the brain require high amounts of thiamine to be able to utilise energy properly. Thiamine is critical to glucose uptake in the brain and as we have seen, if this fuel is running low the brain is far more prone to depression, anxiety and chronic stress. Thiamine is also known to reduce oxidative stress, the wear and tear on cells that is inflammatory to the brain.

Good levels of vitamin B_1 are found in beef and pork, liver, eggs, pulses and nuts. Many grains like rice, wheat, flour and cereals are now fortified, adding thiamine back in after it is lost during processing, although this tends to be with synthetic sources that are poorly absorbed. Good forms of thiamine to look for in supplements are benfotiamine and dibenzoyl thiamine. They are fat soluble, making them more user-friendly for the brain, although water-soluble thiamine is still useful.

Vitamins D_3 + K_2

These are a possible addition to the basic protocol depending on your blood levels. There will usually be some D_3 in a multivitamin, but possibly not enough for your personal needs, so testing is critical.

Vitamin D_3

Actually a pre-hormone, with a similar structure to the sex hormones, vitamin D_3 is a crucial fat-soluble nutrient and it is tough to get enough from foods alone. It is widely acknowledged that vitamin D deficiency is chronic throughout the world and is considered to be the most common medical condition worldwide.

> **GEEK BOX**
>
> **Fat-soluble vitamins**
>
> *There are four fat-soluble vitamins that are essential to our health: vitamins D, K, E and A. Fat soluble means that they get absorbed through the fats in our diet and are stored in fatty tissues in the body. This is why it is important to take vitamins with meals to ensure they are absorbed well. As these vitamins are stored it is possible to have toxic levels, although this is rare and virtually impossible just through diet.*

Vitamin D is essential for many varied functions:

- Immune regulation requires good levels of vitamin D, with low levels making us more suspectable to catching colds, flu and other viral and bacterial infections.
- It supports a healthy balance of many hormones.
- Auto-immune diseases like type 1 diabetes, rheumatoid arthritis and multiple sclerosis are strongly associated with vitamin D deficiency.
- Vitamin D has been shown to help the body fight certain cancers, to benefit the heart and to help regulate blood pressure, and is critically involved in keeping inflammation under control.

Many studies have been done on low vitamin D levels and mental health status. One review study including 31,424 adults found a very strong association between low vitamin D levels and depression. [65]

The big bonus with vitamin D is we can make it ourselves through our skin. Two crucial ingredients are required for this to happen: cholesterol and sunshine. We need adequate cholesterol levels to be able to convert sunshine to vitamin D. Bear in mind that use of sunscreen will stop the manufacture of vitamin D from the sun. Those with darker skin tones need longer exposure but fair skins will burn more easily, so be sensible about the length of time you're in the sun. Many places in the world do not get enough strong sunlight year-round or people may not be getting out in sunshine for long enough, so sunshine is rarely an adequate source of vitamin D.

GEEK BOX

Vitamin D and cholesterol

In order to convert sunshine to vitamin D you need good levels of cholesterol in your skin cells. Vitamin D is later transformed again in the liver and kidneys, but cholesterol is needed for the first step. Low cholesterol can impair how much sunshine is converted to vitamin D. Cholesterol is a critical signalling molecule for the manufacture of steroid hormones such as cortisol, oestrogen and testosterone. It is made largely by the liver (very little comes from the diet). If you get your cholesterol levels checked at the end of winter your LDL is likely to be higher than during the summer, as you haven't been using up the cholesterol for vitamin D production.

There are two forms of dietary vitamin D. Vitamin D_2 is found in mushrooms, especially if they have been exposed to sunlight. You can do this at home simply by placing mushrooms on the windowsill, gills up, for a day or two, allowing levels of vitamin D_2 to greatly increase. Vitamin D_3 is generally considered the more active and bio-available form. It is found in the oily fish wild salmon, trout, tuna, sardines, mackerel and herring; red meat and especially liver; full-fat dairy products; and egg yolks.

Whether obtained from sunshine on the skin, foods or supplements, vitamin D only becomes useful once the liver has converted it to the active form. There are genetic variations that affect how well the liver converts vitamin D, which could be one explanation for why some people naturally maintain optimal levels of vitamin D with little or no supplementation, while others need to take quite high amounts.

Your GP may be happy to run a vitamin D test for you. If not, at-home finger-prick tests are readily available. Symptoms of low mood, poor immune function (being susceptible to infections and slow to fight them off), a craving for sunshine and dreading the dark winter months are good clues that you might be low, but it is always best to test, not guess. Vegans and vegetarians, pregnant women and the very fair-skinned and very dark-skinned tend to be more prone to deficiency, but this is by no means absolute.

GEEK BOX

Optimal vitamin D

Standard reference ranges for vitamin D in the UK are currently 50–200 nmol/L. Below 50 nmol/L is considered deficient. But these ranges are beginning to change and some labs give 50–375 nmol/L, which is a huge sufficiency range. Other reference ranges suggest 75 nmol/L as a minimum. In the US, studies [66] during the Covid-19 pandemic showed that those with higher vitamin D levels fared far better in severity and recovery from the infection, and reported levels above an equivalent of 125 nmol/L to be desirable.

Vitamin K$_2$

Vitamin K$_2$ is another fat-soluble vitamin that is commonly lacking. Found in animal foods, especially red meat, liver and some cheeses, it is also in some fermented foods and recent research suggests that a healthy gut microbiome can produce some vitamin K$_2$.

Vitamin K$_2$ is essential for supporting the body's use of vitamin D$_3$, ensuring the latter gets to where it is needed. The two combined help to integrate calcium into the bones rather than its being dumped in joints and blood vessels. Vitamin K$_2$ is critical for healthy blood clotting and supports healthy immune regulation. It appears to help with blood glucose regulation, which in turn influences mood disorders.

Taking a supplement containing vitamin K_2 along with vitamin D_3 may be advisable, especially if you find you are low in vitamin D and your level is slow to improve with just a D_3 supplement. They are often found together in pill or spray form. The dose will depend on your test results, but take with food and ideally in the morning. The theory behind this is simply that the body associates bursts of vitamin D with sun exposure, so mimic that by providing vitamin D at a time when the sun is high in the sky. Recommended levels are hugely variable and should be determined by your blood test.

Omega 3 fish oil

As we saw in Chapter Six, the brain is roughly 60% fat, with around 20% of these fats omega 3 fatty acids, which are found largely in the grey matter of the brain and serve many functions to keep it healthy. The development of neurons, maintenance of a healthy myelin sheath (which coats the nerves) and regulation of other processes throughout the brain all depend on these essential fats. Our brain cannot be healthy without adequate omega 3 and the body cannot make these fatty acids itself, so we have to get them from our food on a regular basis.

Scientific evidence on the beneficial impact of omega 3 supplementation on anxiety and depression varies, with some studies showing significant improvements with consistent use of 1000 mg of fish oil daily, while other studies are inconclusive, so more research is required. One study on patients with major depressive disorder unresponsive to treatment did conclude that *'low omega 3 levels caused antidepressants to work less well'*. [67,68,69]

However, the benefits to overall brain health of increased omega 3 levels are pretty conclusive, from Parkinson's to Alzheimer's, attention deficit disorder to schizophrenia and autism. The mechanism of the brain benefit from omega 3 is mostly to do with it helping communication between brain cells, aiding in brain chemical balance, as well as its strong anti-inflammatory effect leading to lower levels of inflammation in the brain. There are studies reporting reduced aggression and anti-social behaviours in adult offenders in prison when they supplement with omega 3. Moreover, omega 3 fatty acids are believed to help improve the integrity of the gut lining, reducing the risk of a leaky gut.

Omega 3 fatty acids come in different structures, long chain and short chain. The short-chain omega 3s are found in plant sources like flax, hemp, chia and walnuts, but it is the long-chain omega 3s that the brain needs. It is possible for the body to convert short chain to long chain, but only inefficiently, with just a small percentage of the short-chain omega 3 we eat being turned into the important long-chain form. Due to genetics and other factors like gut health, some people can't make this conversion at all. The best food sources for long-chain omega 3s are oily fish. Ensuring adequate consumption of the right type of fish is therefore imperative and if your diet is not rich in oily fish, supplementing is wise.

The quality of a fish oil supplement is very important. Omega 3 fatty acids are extremely vulnerable to being damaged through exposure to light, oxygen and heat, so creating a supplement without causing harm to them is a tricky and relatively expensive business. Look on the label for terms such as 'cold water, low pressure distillation', 'no solvents' or 'clean and stable'. You shouldn't get a strong fishy smell when you open the pot or get fishy burps after taking fish oil capsules. If you do, it could be that the product has turned rancid, rendering the omega 3s not only no longer good for you but potentially harmful.

If you choose not to consume animal products or if you have an allergy to fish, there is a good supplement solution in the form of a special type of microalgae. These plant marine algae are grown specifically for this purpose in controlled environments to avoid contaminants. They provide omega 3 in the ready-to-go long-chain form, the difference to fish oils being they have a different ratio of the two main therapeutic components, EPA and DHA (see Geek Box). An algae supplement (often referred to as vegan omega 3) is a sustainable option due to over-fishing in much of the world. But do buy a good-quality brand and check that the source is from algae, not flax seeds.

CAUTION: Those on blood-thinning medications need to check with their prescribing doctor before taking fish oil supplements, as omega 3s thin the blood so your medication may need to be adjusted.

GEEK BOX

Omega 3 fatty acids

Omega 3 fatty acids come in three forms: ALA (alpha-linolenic acid), EPA (eicosapentaenoic acid) and DHA (docosahexaenoic acid). Plant forms contain only ALA, which is a precursor to EPA and DHA, meaning that ALA can be converted from the short-chain form to the long-chain forms. However, the conversion of ALA to EPA and DHA is inefficient. High levels of many nutrients are required to make this conversion, including magnesium, zinc, iron, calcium, copper and some of the B vitamins. Plant foods are low in many of these nutrients, making the conversion rate of ALA even lower in vegetarians and vegans. The condition of the digestive system and certain genetic factors can also determine how much is converted, making it almost impossible to know how much EPA and DHA someone is able to make from ALA. This is where testing can be helpful.

There are health benefits to omega 3 in the ALA form. Some studies suggest it can have a beneficial influence on the balance of LDL and HDL cholesterol in the blood and a possible lowering effect of triglycerides and blood pressure, plus foods high in ALA like flax, hemp and chia seeds have many additional benefits when eaten as whole seeds (see Chapter Six).

EPA and DHA are the long-chain form that is readily used by the body. These are found in animal fats like oily fish, egg yolks and grass-fed meat, as well as a specific type of algae – the only non-animal form. EPA is a crucial part of inflammation management, with potent anti-inflammatory benefits. Hence it is associated with improved heart and vascular health as well as a healthy brain. DHA is found in high amounts in the eye and brain. Low levels, especially in childhood, are associated with cognitive impairment.

Testing for omega 3 can be helpful, as individual differences make it impossible to know if the amount in someone's diet is adequate and, if not, what degree of supplementation is required. Some people are genetically more prone to inflammation, making their need greater, and some genetic types make it harder to use omega 3 from food. A blood test can also show your omega 6:3 ratio, which is a useful guide to your food or supplement need. It is easy to consume too much omega 6 from vegetable and seed oils, processed foods high in these oils and products from animals fed on grains not grass. It is widely accepted that the ideal ratio of omega 6:3 should be around 2:1, meaning there is twice the amount of omega 6 to omega 3 in your body. A ratio of 20:1 is commonly found in those who eat a standard Westernised diet, so much more effort needs to be put in to get adequate omega 3 into the system.

It has recently become easier and far cheaper to get tested privately, and some GPs will also test for omega 3 and 6 if asked. Getting your omega 6:3 ratio tested before supplementing and then after a year of supplementation will give a clear indication of whether the supplement you are taking is being utilised by your body. It is important to wait at least a year as it takes time for the tissues to replace omega 6 with omega 3.

Magnesium

Known as the master mineral, magnesium works in many ways throughout the body and brain. It has an influence on over 600 cellular reactions, in particular calming the stress response, blood pressure regulation, nerve and muscle function, bone health and integrity of the blood–brain barrier, helping to protect the brain from toxins. Common symptoms of low magnesium are fatigue, low mood, irritability and inability to relax. Many digestive problems and blood sugar issues can be helped with higher levels of magnesium.

Low levels of magnesium can affect one's ability to absorb vitamin D. A combined lack of magnesium and vitamin D greatly increases the risk of depression, anxiety and other mental health disorders. Magnesium is also a huge player in the regulation of the nervous system, helping calm the over-revving of too much stress, downregulating the excitatory systems in the brain and helping to activate vagal tone, supporting digestion, sleep and recovery.

Magnesium is found in many whole foods, but due to chronic depletion in the soil and loss of magnesium due to modern food processing, levels are far lower than they used to be. Dairy foods, fish and dark chocolate are great sources, as are nuts, especially almonds and cashews; beans, especially black beans and soy beans; flax seeds and pumpkin seeds; oats, green vegetables and bananas. We do need high levels of magnesium so the quality of food sources is important: opt for minimally processed foods that look as close to the way they do in nature as possible.

Magnesium is very unstable and needs to be attached to something else, also known as chelated, to make it useful to the body. The amount contained in a supplement can be misleading as there is the elemental amount, the actual amount of magnesium, and then the amount of elemental magnesium in combination with whatever it's been mixed with, usually an amino acid like glycine or taurine (see Geek Box). Good-quality supplements tend to list both the elemental and the total magnesium. If only the total is listed you have no idea how much actual magnesium you are getting. There are different benefits depending on what the magnesium is mixed with.

GEEK BOX

Forms of magnesium

With so many different forms of magnesium in supplements, the devil is in the detail.

- *Cheap forms such as magnesium oxide and magnesium chloride tend to stay in the digestive system and have a relaxing effect on the bowels. This can be helpful for constipation, which in itself is associated with poor mental health.*
- *To get adequate magnesium into the brain, the magnesium needs*

to be able to pass from the digestive tract into the blood and then up into the brain, passing the gut barrier and then across the blood–brain barrier. There is one form of magnesium that is readily taken up by the brain, magnesium threonate, but it is very pricey. Two other forms are well absorbed through the gut wall and are believed to get into the brain – magnesium glycinate (or bisglycinate) and magnesium taurate – and these are far more affordable.

- For stress and sleep support as well as a happy brain, magnesium glycinate comes out on top. The glycine greatly improves the absorption of the magnesium into the brain. Glycine is another inhibitory nutrient, calming the over-revving of the brain; it helps with sleep quality through its brain-calming functions and helping the body cool down at night, while also reducing night-time urination. Glycine can also help with balancing insulin, blood glucose levels and burning body fat, which in turn reduces inflammation and helps our brain balance better. Without enough glycine we can't make sufficient cell-protecting glutathione, the master antioxidant important for the health of all our cells, especially our brain cells, which are so vulnerable to being harmed by oxidative stress. Glycine is in a lot of foods but getting it into the brain on the back of magnesium is a great way to optimise the benefits of both.
- Magnesium taurate has taurine, a different amino acid, attached to it. Taurine is also calming, neuroprotective and anti-inflammatory for the brain. It helps with stress, relaxation and sleep as well as heart health and blood pressure, and is discussed further in the special supplements section.

The vast majority of the magnesium in our body is inside our cells, so testing for magnesium in blood (serum) is not particularly helpful. By the time serum levels are low, the cells will be desperately low. Some doctors will test for red blood cell (RBC) levels of magnesium, which gives a more accurate indication of your body's stores. It is often worthwhile to take a good-quality magnesium supplement, with food, for a few weeks and see if symptoms improve rather than relying on blood tests.

Specialist supplements

So that's the basic supplement protocol for a happy brain: a good multivitamin and mineral, possibly an additional methylated B complex, D_3 + K_2, omega 3 fish oil and magnesium glycinate at night. This suits most people and covers most needs.

This section explains some further supplements you might want to consider. Use this information as guidance to equip you with knowledge and strategic questions that you can ask a registered nutritionist or other natural health professional to see if you might benefit from adding one or some of these nutrients to your daily routine. Remember, food first is always the best option. Supplements can only be helpful in addition to a healthy diet.

Vitamin C: Antioxidant, immune supporter, happy gut promoter

Vitamin C is readily found in a lot of foods that many people are eating on a daily basis, so supplementation might be deemed unnecessary. However, as is often the case, studies on depressed patients tend to show low levels and greater need. Very low levels are associated with scurvy, which causes deep fatigue and bone deformity, but most people benefit from additional vitamin C well above what is considered adequate to avoid disease.

Vitamin C has many functions throughout the body:

- It is a key player in the immune system, is supportive of our cardiovascular function and appears to help keep our arteries clear of plaque, likely due to its strong antioxidant capacity, protecting our insides from oxidative damage. Without adequate vitamin C we can struggle to absorb enough iron

from our food, a major risk factor in depression.
- It assists in gut microbial diversity and protects the gut lining from becoming too 'leaky', both essential for a happy gut. Collagen, a protein that keeps skin, muscles bone, hair, nails and the gut lining healthy and strong, also requires vitamin C to work properly.
- Vitamin C is involved in the regulation of certain neurotransmitters, in particular dopamine and serotonin, and is important in the management of those excitatory chemicals that can drive feelings of anxiety and overwhelm. As a potent antioxidant, vitamin C is also important for protecting the brain from damage and inflammation. Patients with depression tend to have increased levels of oxidative stress, resulting in a greater need for antioxidants.
- The adrenal glands, which sit on top of our kidneys and make adrenaline and cortisol, our main stress hormones, require far more vitamin C than any other part of the human body. People who are depressed and anxious tend to have higher stress levels. If your vitamin C supply is being hijacked by your adrenal demand, that could leave you running low in the brain.

We cannot make or store vitamin C, so it's very important to get some at every meal. Kiwi fruits, red and orange peppers, citrus fruits and leafy greens are all great sources, but virtually all plant foods contain some vitamin C. As it is water soluble, levels greatly reduce if foods are cooked in water, so either save the cooking water for making soups or stews or steam your veggies to preserve the vitamin C content.

Most multivitamins and minerals contain a small amount of vitamin C. It is also available separately in powder or pill form, mostly sold as ascorbic acid. Dose tolerance is very individual but in general 1000 mg, taken with food, is safe and well tolerated. Increase the dose gradually to avoid an upset stomach or diarrhoea.

Curcumin: An anti-inflammatory superstar

Curcumin is a gut-friendly polyphenol and one of many bioactive compounds found in the spicy root turmeric. In recent decades many studies have been conducted to try to understand why this spice has so many health-giving properties.

- One of the main benefits appears to be its ability to reduce inflammation via various routes, including better management of insulin. As explained in Chapter Two, good blood sugar management is fundamental to good mental health. Curcumin acts as an antioxidant to help mitigate some of the damage caused by oxidative stress, while also helping to redress the insulin resistance itself.
- Another cause of inflammation in the brain is exposure to toxins, from the environment or from within the body. A leaky gut (discussed in Chapter Three) can result in highly inflammatory by-products of gut bacteria called lipopolysaccharides (LPS) passing from the gut into the blood and up to the brain. Curcumin not only helps calm the damage of LPS in the brain, it tightens up the cells of the gut to stop the leaky gut happening in the first place.
- Curcumin has balancing effects on the stress hormone cortisol, an excess of which in the brain is inflammatory. Studies have shown that curcumin has alleviated depressive and other psychological alterations induced by excess cortisol. [70]
- Curcumin stimulates production of BDNF (see Chapters Four and Five), which helps keep the brain capable of learning and renewing neural pathways and is further associated with a reduction of depressive symptoms.
- Curcumin slows the breakdown of the neurotransmitter acetylcholine, one of the major regulators of brain chemistry.
- Curcumin has also been shown in animal studies to alter

levels of the neurotransmitters serotonin and dopamine while calming the overstimulation of glutamate, which then allows for greater levels of calming GABA to be taken up into the brain. This neurotransmitter-balancing action of curcumin is thought to be acting in similar ways to SSRIs and other anti-depressant and anti-anxiety medications, although they are not interchangeable. Do consult with your prescribing healthcare professional before taking curcumin.

Incorporating turmeric into your meals is a great way to provide tiny doses of curcumin and combining it with fats and other spices, especially black pepper, can help your body absorb it better. Turmeric has been part of Asian cooking for millennia and is still used in many Eastern diets daily, but if you don't eat curries and other spiced foods frequently, consuming enough to produce a therapeutic benefit requires supplementation.

Turmeric supplements used to be considered ineffective because absorption of bioactive curcumin is very poor. Recent advances in supplement technologies have seen various solutions, including adding piperine, a substance found in black pepper (and therefore present in many traditional dishes where turmeric and black pepper feature together); creating a liposomal version, meaning it is suspended in tiny fat particles, making it much more bio-available; and other developments that make the curcumin 'cell active' and critically able to cross the blood–brain barrier. These supplements are more expensive than standard turmeric or curcumin supplements due to the added expense of creating a highly absorbable product, but it's definitely worth it.

Curcumin is generally well tolerated, although starting slowly is advisable as some people can get an upset stomach with high levels. This is mostly due to poor quality and therefore poor absorption. Don't take it on an empty stomach for this reason and to help absorption. Also, curcumin is known to block iron absorption, so if you are prone to anaemia or low iron, be cautious about taking curcumin and don't take it at the same time as iron supplements or iron-rich foods.

MCT oil: Readily available brain fuel

MCT (medium-chain triglyceride) oil is a concentrate from coconut oil, which converts into ketones very readily. Ketones are naturally produced by the body when it's in fat-burning mode, providing quick, clean fuel for the body and brain. Almost all our cells, including brain cells, can run on glucose or ketones, but if, as explored in Chapter Two, your brain prefers ketones, and/or if it can't manage its glucose supply very well, then provision of ketones is going to make a huge difference to how your brain functions and how you feel mentally and physically.

MCT oil does what your body fat should be doing, providing fuel in the form of ketones when glucose is not available. Using MCT oil is thus ideal to help you through the adaptation period of making long-term dietary and lifestyle changes that will facilitate your body readily burning your body fat, providing you with a steady supply of ketones naturally.

Take between 1 teaspoon and 1 tablespoon of MCT oil several times a day. It's best to take it as soon as you notice a drop in in mental or physical energy, are craving sugar or are beginning to get anxious for no obvious reason. Take it off the spoon like a medicine or add it to food or drinks. It is odourless and tasteless.

Buy MCT oil that is 80–100% C8 (caprylic acid). This is the form most easily used by your brain.

Choline (citicoline): The brain booster

Choline is an essential nutrient that is similar to the B vitamins and has many roles in the body's metabolic and brain-balancing systems. It is a nootropic, meaning it enhances brain function. It converts to acetylcholine, a neurotransmitter that influences levels of serotonin and dopamine, which have been shown to be low in depressed and anxious patients. Choline is neuroprotective, likely due to its anti-inflammatory and antioxidant properties. It also supports mitochondrial energy production and vagal tone, promoting relaxation and reduced anxiety while helping to increase focus and alertness.

> *In a study of 50 patients on antidepressants the addition of a special form of choline, citicoline, to the anti-depressant medication saw an improvement in symptoms and speed of recovery.* [71]

Many foods contain choline, especially liver, chicken, fish and pulses. It is quite easy to consume adequate choline, but as we age we use it less well.

Citicoline or CDP-choline is a specific form of choline that is readily used by the brain and is the most effective form for supplementation. It has been found to be very safe to take, even at high levels, with the only possible side effect being some digestive disturbance, although this is rare and quickly resolved when levels are reduced. The dose is key. Supplements usually contain 250–500 mg, but some people find doses as high as 2000 mg are required. Start slowly and monitor any changes you notice in brain energy, concentration and mood stability.

L-Taurine: The GABA-friendly amino acid

Taurine is a non-essential amino acid, meaning we can make it in the body using other amino acids, but as we age we do this less well. Taurine supplementation has long been used to help with migraines, menstrual issues, sleep and anxiety. Taurine's effect on anxiety is thanks to its calming effect in the brain, similar to GABA and glycine. Research has found that low levels of taurine could accelerate ageing and increase the likelihood of high blood glucose and diabetes, abdominal obesity, high blood pressure and fatty liver disease, all chronic conditions associated with the modern ageing process. [72] As all these conditions are also systemically inflammatory, and inflammation in the brain is a known cause or accelerator of poor mental health, this is an important finding.

Taurine is mostly found in animal foods, meat, fish and dairy. Taking taurine as a supplement may be especially worth considering if you eat a mostly or entirely plant-based diet. Taurine supplements can be taken during the day (500–2000 mg) for help with anxiety and with magnesium glycinate (200–400 mg) at night to support better sleep and brain health.

L-Theanine: The anxiety super-supplement

Theanine is another very calming amino acid. It is well studied for its benefits in healthy brain ageing and is especially useful for those prone to anxiety and overwhelm. Its beneficial action comes from calming the stress hormone cortisol in the brain, while blocking excess glutamic acid, which can be overly excitatory. This enables greater production of the calming brain chemical GABA. Theanine can also boost levels of serotonin. Brain scans have shown that it increases levels of the slower, calmer alpha brain waves, as seen in those who are meditating.

Theanine takes 40–60 minutes to have an effect. Taken before a morning coffee it can help cognition and focus and balance the stimulation of caffeine. For a racing or ruminating mind at night it can be taken an hour before bedtime and is a calming, soothing and sleep-promoting combination with magnesium glycinate.

Theanine is found in green and black tea, especially green matcha tea, which is likely why people who are caffeine sensitive can tolerate tea better than coffee. Two cups of green tea can be mood boosting. However, levels of theanine in tea can vary greatly, so supplementation is much more reliable.

A standard supplement dose is around 200 mg, although far higher levels have been found to be safe and effective for some people. As with all supplements, start low and slow and take note of any changes you experience.

5-HTP: The depression super-supplement

CAUTION: Do not take 5-HTP if you are using anti-depressant medications.

The compound 5-HTP (5-hydroxytryptophan), extracted from the African plant *Griffonia simplicifolia*, is well studied as an alternative to anti-depressant medication. Tryptophan is an essential amino acid, meaning we can't make it so we must consume it, and is the main precursor ingredient required to make serotonin and melatonin in the brain. It has therapeutic benefit for people with depression, anxiety and insomnia and can also be helpful for migraine sufferers.

We can get some tryptophan from eating poultry, eggs, pumpkin seeds and dairy foods. However, levels in food tend to be low. For a more therapeutic effect, supplementation is generally required.

There are very few side effects of 5-HTP supplements, most commonly nausea or other stomach upset, although this is rare at the recommended dosage. As around 90% of the serotonin in the body is made in the gut, this could explain why some people experience digestive problems. It is important to take 5-HTP on an empty stomach otherwise the tryptophan will have to compete with other more abundant amino acids in your food and will not be able to make it up to the brain. Dosage varies a lot depending on age, reason for use and other medications, so do get professional advice before taking 5-HTP.

Inositol: The missing B vitamin

Inositol used to be called vitamin B_8. It is very calming, greatly helps with an anxious, overly busy brain and regulates neurotransmitters to relieve depression. It is found in the central nervous system, which allows our nerves to communicate throughout the body and brain. Many studies have shown improvements in the brain's GABA management after supplementation with inositol, helping decrease agitation and increasing calm while also improving serotonin management. The inositol levels of depressed and suicidal patients have been shown to be lower than average.

> *Inositol was found to be more effective than antidepressants for some anxiety sufferers, especially those who experience panic attacks.* [73]

Other benefits of inositol are experienced in menstrual and metabolic dysregulation including polycystic ovary syndrome (PCOS), premenstrual syndrome (PMS), insulin resistance/high blood glucose, high blood pressure and poor cholesterol management. If taken at night, inositol can be very helpful for better sleep.

Some plant foods contain inositol but levels are low, making it hard to get enough for therapeutic benefit.

Myo-inositol is the specific form of inositol to supplement with. It is safe to take in general and alongside psychiatric medication. It can work incredibly well for some people and only marginally or not at all for others. The dose starts at around 4 g, but doses as high as 18 g a day are considered safe; studies have used 12 g a day in split doses for depressed patients. It is far easier to use as a powder dissolved in water rather than in pill form, especially if taking higher doses. Seek advice from a clinical nutritionist or medical practitioner for the best dose for your particular requirements.

Lithium orotate: The missing mineral

Lithium is calming for the brain thanks to its neuroprotective and neurotransmitter-balancing effects and it increases BDNF, the nourishing repair molecule the brain needs to thrive.

Lithium can increase levels of oxytocin, boosting feelings of connection and love while reducing fear.

Lithium is a mineral that exists in the earth's crust and is in the water supply and is found at low levels in some foods, mostly grains and vegetables. Naturally occurring levels vary greatly around the world, but the average natural dose from food and water is around 2–5 mg a day.

> ***Studies have shown that geographical areas with low lithium have much higher rates of depression than places with naturally high levels.***

Lithium in the form of lithium carbonate or lithium citrate is given as a psychiatric medication to patients with mania and bipolar disorder, but **this is not what is being recommended here.** Lithium orotate is sold over the counter as a supplement and is used for blood glucose and insulin regulation as well as in mood and depressive disorders. It is important to appreciate that lithium orotate doses are tiny compared to those used in medications. Where a prescription drug might contain 1000–1800 mg of lithium, supplementation generally starts at 5 mg. This is about the level naturally present in a wholefood, natural diet.

Lithium orotate supplementation is not something that is recommended over the long term. The benefits are generally felt very quickly. Once you have restored your cellular levels, stopping or going down to micro doses of around 300 mcg is advisable. You can top up again on a cyclical basis to ensure your levels remain optimal. Seek professional guidance from a clinical nutritionist or medical practitioner.

Berberine: The metabolic and gut–brain heavy hitter

Berberine is a natural compound found in goldenseal and Oregon grape and has been used for thousands of years in traditional Chinese medicine. It helps in insulin and blood glucose regulation and subsequent improvements in burning fat and making ketones. In fact, it is often cited as being clinically as effective as metformin, one of the main medications for type 2 diabetics.

Berberine is also a natural anti-pathogen for the gut, killing off bad bugs and yeasts and supporting beneficial bugs to help them thrive, including those all-important butyrate-producing gut microbes.[74] Studies have shown that regular intake of berberine improves cholesterol levels, heart health and blood pressure. More recently berberine has been looked at for its anti-depressive potential. Although not fully understood yet, it appears to help reduce neuroinflammation, promotes the growth of neurons and seems to positively modulate neurotransmitter balance.[75]

Berberine is mostly found in 500 mg capsules. Ideally take it 30 minutes before a meal for its glucose- and insulin-regulating properties (but if you forget take it at the beginning of the meal), 2–3 times a day. Berberine should not be taken long term. Try it for eight weeks and then have a break.

Medicinal mushrooms: The future of brain health?

Eating mushrooms on a regular basis is a great way to get a potent prebiotic fibre called beta-glucans, plus vitamin D_2 and copper, a very important mineral for a healthy, happy brain. All mushrooms contain these beneficial compounds in varying amounts. They also contain the master antioxidant glutathione and a lesser-known antioxidant called ergothioneine, a brain booster and anti-inflammatory. The culinary mushrooms with the highest levels of ergothioneine are porcini, followed by king oyster, maitake, oyster and shiitake. Cooking them does not destroy their medicinal properties. Sautéed in butter or olive oil with some garlic, they make a nutritious happy brain side dish.

Medicinal mushrooms have higher concentrations of these and many, many more compounds shown to help with gut health, brain health, immune and hormonal regulation. Unlike most medications that work on singular pathways in the body, medicinal mushrooms work in a network of ways, much like they do in nature where they can communicate over thousands of miles to manage the health of many plant and fungal species. This level of sophistication and adaptability is essential for supporting human health, where there are often many factors at play.

The quality and extract concentration of medicinal mushrooms are of the utmost importance, as you can end up spending a lot of money on products that are not providing any real benefit due to poor extraction processes or simply not enough of the active ingredients being present. It's worth consulting a specialist to get the correct types and strengths for your needs. Medicinal mushrooms are better absorbed when vitamin C is present but away from other foods, so take them first thing in the morning, with some lemon water if vitamin C has not been added to your particular capsules.

Some happy brain medical mushrooms to consider are the following:

- **Lion's mane** is a powerful anti-inflammatory and antioxidant, a favourite for gut health, cognition and brain health. Lion's mane has been clinically proven to regulate cellular brain health by increasing BDNF and nerve growth factor levels, which support concentration, processing speed and memory while also improving mood regulation. Lion's mane also has a calming effect on the brain as it contains GABA. One study concluded that there was a clinically measurable improvement in symptoms of depression and anxiety in 30 women who were given lion's mane for four weeks as compared to placebo. [76]
- **Reishi** is used for energy balance and stress hormone support; for people struggling with low energy, thyroid disorders, adrenal exhaustion and anxiety disorders; and to improve sleep quality. It has anti-inflammatory and neuroprotective properties. A combination of lion's mane and reishi is a great blend to help with depression, gut dysbiosis and energy issues. Combining these highly complex organisms creates an even more complex and synergistic effect.

- **Cordyceps** has been shown in research [77] to help an over-stressed mind and body and to support good-quality sleep as well as immune regulation and energy production. Like reishi it is apoptogenic, helping regulate the nervous system.

Herbs

Many herbal remedies have been used in traditional medicine as mood and mental health tonics. It is impossible to know which might suit you best, but the herbs listed here are safe, well researched and worth trying. Many supplemental tinctures and powdered blends contain a mixture of herbs, which may provide greater benefit.

- **Valerian**, nature's Valium, helps calm an anxious brain due to its ability to increase GABA, while also regulating serotonin levels, helping sleep and depressive disorders.
- **Chamomile** is commonly used as a calming night-time tea and is included in many sleep aids. Its main active compound is apigenin, a muscle relaxant, gentle sedative, antioxidant, anti-inflammatory and neuroprotective. Apigenin is also now available as a supplement.
- **Passionflower** is known to increase levels of GABA in the brain, helping with anxiety and sleep.
- *Bacopa monnieri* (water hyssop) and **gotu kola** (*Centella asiatica*) are two herbs that have been well researched for their use in cognitive decline and memory issues through improving acetylcholine levels in the brain. This same mechanism can greatly enhance mood and depression. Gotu kola also improves blood circulation, increasing delivery of nutrients and oxygen to the brain.
- **Marshmallow root** and **slippery elm** are both great for feeding the gut microbes and for calming inflammation. Marshmallow root also provides plenty of prebiotic fibre (see the next section).

- Saffron has been widely studied in animals and to a lesser degree in humans for its anti-depressant benefits. Clinical trials have found greater benefit for patients with depression and anxiety from saffron over conventional medications:

   Active biological compounds [in saffron] ... play a pivotal role in the central nervous system associated with anxiety and depression ... saffron was as effective as chemically derived antidepressants such as fluoxetine in mild to moderate depression [and] was equally effective as citalopram in major depressive disorder with anxious distress and decreased mild to moderate generalized anxiety disorder when compared with sertraline. [78]

Prebiotics and probiotics

Getting plenty of prebiotic fibre to feed your happy gut microbes by eating more plant-based foods and freshening them up with some living fermented foods is always the best option – food first! See Chapters Five and Six for more on this. However, pre- and probiotic supplements can be a great addition to make up for gaps and challenges in your diet and lifestyle due to travel, lack of time, personal taste and food availability.

Prebiotic fibre

Since modern diets are often lacking in amounts and types of fibre, a prebiotic powder is a quick and easy way to supercharge your microbial families. One of our keystone microbes, *Akkermansia muciniphila*, is especially partial to these fibres and if fed prebiotics regularly gives back in many healthful and happy brain ways. *Akkermansia* is an important master strain gut microbe that communicates with the other gut microbes, helping to manage the healthy composition and function of the gut microbiome. It is also instrumental in keeping the gut wall healthy, which helps avoid leaky gut and all the inflammatory issues this can cause.

Prebiotic use is increasingly being seen as a safe and highly effective strategy for maintaining good gut health and supporting metabolic function. If you want to try a prebiotic fibre, look for one with a range of different prebiotic ingredients, rather than just one, as it's impossible to know the exact types of fibre you will benefit from most.

For some people these concentrated fibres can initially cause some bloating. This is usually due to the numbers or types of microbes being a little suboptimal. Cut down to very small amounts and raise them slowly. This will give your gut microbes time to adjust and increase in number without overwhelming your system.

Types of prebiotic fibre to look out for include the following:

- **Inulin**, a type of fibre that gut bugs really love, is found in onions, garlic, leeks, Jerusalem artichokes, green/greenish bananas (they need to be only just becoming yellow, otherwise the inulin is turning to sugar) and asparagus. It is now readily available as a powder that you can add to foods and drinks. Start slowly.
- **FOS** (fructooligosaccharides) are a gentler option for those who find inulin too activating (bloating and wind). They are readily found in the allium family (garlic, onions, etc.), asparagus, tomatoes and other fruits, notably green bananas, plus many vegetables including sea vegetables like seaweed. FOS are also available as a supplement.
- **GOS** (galactooligosaccharides) are found in high amounts in Jerusalem artichokes and in lesser amounts in lentils and butter/lima beans. Again, this type of prebiotic is often found in supplement powders.
- **PHGG** (partially hydrolysed guar gum) is extracted from the guar bean and is not something you're likely to be eating much of. It's a great one to supplement with as its prebiotic benefits are well established.

- **Potato starch** is a great prebiotic resistant starch. It can be produced by cooking potatoes and cooling them for at least six hours (you can then reheat them). Some of the normal starch changes structure during this process, becoming resistant to your digestion and a superfood for your gut microbes (see Chapter Five). Powdered potato starch is readily available.
- **Apple pectin** is found in whole apples, especially in and just beneath the skin, and in higher amounts in green and sour apples. Pectin is also found in the pith of citrus fruits and both are great prebiotic sources. Apple pectin can also be bought in supplement form.

Probiotics

Despite the differing views and controversy about what can help alleviate depression and anxiety, what is very clear, as I have stressed throughout this book, is that a happy brain relies on a happy gut. A happy gut requires lots and lots of beneficial gut microbes known as probiotics (pro-life). Eating a wide range of live fermented foods is consistently touted as one of the very best ways to enhance gut health, so do what you can to include a range of live foods day to day (there are suggestions on how to do this in Chapters Five and Six).

Eating a varied, colourful, high-fibre diet that includes some fermented foods is often adequate, but you may want to supercharge your gut microbes by supplementing with probiotics. This is especially useful during and following times of chronic stress, travel, medication use or maybe even a run of poor-quality food. It also fine to simply take some probiotic supplements occasionally throughout the year to top up your own beneficial microbes.

Possible benefits of taking a probiotic supplement for mental health include:

- Systemic reduction of inflammation, a well-known trigger for many mental health issues
- Improved vagal tone, creating a stronger bi-directional signalling pathway between brain and gut
- Reduction in stress hormones, allowing for better sleep and a less anxious response to life's stressors
- Increased BDNF, keeping the brain fit and healthy
- Improved nutrient absorption, including omega 3 fatty acid uptake in the brain
- Beneficial gut microbes helping to crowd out and keep at bay pathogenic microbes, which are associated with depression and anxiety

Creating a functional probiotic product has a lot of challenges. First, how do you keep bacteria alive throughout production where they get capsulated, then sit in a warehouse and then on a shop shelf before finally ending up being consumed by the customer? Even if this problem is overcome, the live bacteria's next challenge is to get through the very hostile, high-acid environment of the stomach (which is designed to kill bugs) and then roughly 6 metres of small intestine before reaching their final destination in the large intestine. Many companies put in vast numbers of beneficial microbes, far more than advertised on the label, to allow for some die-off. Enteric-coated supplements have been developed to protect the delicate live bacteria from the acid once in the stomach and providers often recommend consuming probiotics on an empty stomach when stomach acid levels are generally far lower to further support their viability. Some probiotic supplements are in spore form, making them far more robust.

There are two main families of bacterial species you will see on labels: *Lactobacillus* (often shortened to L.) and *Bifidobacterium* (B.). This family is the genus and is followed by the species, then sometimes a set of numbers, which is the specific strain. Look for a product that contains a range of these strains. The producers are not allowed to state specific benefits unless clinically proven, so the label can only hint at what a certain probiotic might help with, not make any health claims.

There is a vast range of probiotic supplements. However, it has become increasingly clear that taking large numbers of random strains of bacteria is a rather hit-and-miss approach and is not recommended. More targeted probiotic use, looking at how specific strains work for different health issues, is still in its infancy. For now, it's best to go by your symptoms. If you take a probiotic and you feel better – for instance, your bloating, constipation or diarrhoea improves – then it's likely a good one for you. Alternatively, look for a product that contains at least some of these strains, as they have been clinically researched for their use in patients with anxiety and depression:

- *Bifidobacterium longum* 1714™ improves the use of tryptophan in the process of making serotonin and melatonin.
- *B. longum* 04 lowers cortisol and decreases symptoms in patients with anxiety and depression.
- *L. helveticus* lowers cortisol and neuroinflammation, and decreases symptoms in patients with anxiety and depression. Found in Emmental and other Swiss cheeses.
- *L.. helveticus* Rosell®-52 + *B. longum* Rosell®-175 may improve social anxiety and depressive symptoms.
- *L. plantarum* may help increase serotonin and dopamine and decrease cortisol. Good for IBS. Found in some fermented vegetables.
- *L. rhamnosus* lowers anxiety by increasing GABA after about six weeks. Found in some live yogurts.
- *L. reuteri* lowers anxiety through increased GABA production and reduces inflammation and cortisol.
- *L. fermentum* is very helpful for those who have taken antibiotics. Found in some fermented vegetables.

If you feel bloated or have bowel disturbances while taking a probiotic, reduce or stop the dose and try again on a lower dose more slowly once things have normalised for you. If you continue to react it's worth trying a different product, but keep what you have as you may tolerate it in the future once you've worked on your gut microbes with other diet and lifestyle support.

CHAPTER NINE
Live Your Brain Happy

So far in the happy brain action plan we've looked at what we eat and drink and how we can make changes and add boosters to improve the nutrients we provide for our body and brain. But it's not all about food – there are plenty of other happy brain hacks that can be transformative in the management of anxiety and depression. It's these lifestyle changes that this chapter explores.

As with making changes to your diet, start gently and see what fits comfortably for you. Once you find one tool that feels doable daily and appears to be bringing you benefit, keep going until it becomes an effortless habit. You can then come back to the list and choose something else to add to your toolkit.

There is no right or wrong, no one approach that is better than any other. Be open to change, be curious about how these practices are reprogramming the old wiring of your brain that was keeping you stuck, and move on if you begin to feel frustrated or defeated by the process. Trying again after you've made dietary and other lifestyle changes may well make something that feels impossibly difficult today far easier and attainable in a few weeks or months.

Vagus nerve stimulation

As you may remember from Chapter Four, the vagus nerve is the superhighway to good gut–brain communication. This bi-directional flow of instructions, feedback and sensory signals is what makes us human. Take a moment to really think about this. Your brain is constantly receiving intelligence from internal and external cues. If your nervous system is overly activated, triggering a danger response at the slightest concern or challenge, your brain will do exactly as it should: prepare you for fight or flight by actioning the stress hormones and driving up your anxiety. The brain isn't faulty, it's the messaging that's incorrect. Similarly, if your brain is being told there is not enough fuel and a lack of critical nutrients to go around, it will do what it needs to: dial down your metabolism both mentally and physically.

The vagus nerve is what relays many of these neural prompts to the brain from the information being put out by your gut microbes and gut-based immune system. It is 'listening in' to what is going on between these two highly intelligent sensing systems and then shooting the latest news up to the brain in a fraction of a second to keep it in the loop.

> *A recent study looking at vagus nerve function not only confirmed that healthy gut microbes have a positive effect on mood via the vagus nerve's communication system, but also that they improve the action of anti-depressant drugs (SSRIs) on mood.* [79]

Stress is kryptonite to the vagus nerve, meaning most of us have to get better at calming and soothing our nervous system to allow more of our innate restoration processes to be activated. As is so often the way, there's no absolute to what works best for everyone. It's trial and error, so experiment to find out the methods to stimulate the vagus nerve that are easiest for you to implement most often.

GEEK BOX

HeartMath

HeartMath® offers fantastic training to anyone wanting to learn skills to manage stress and activate the vagus nerve. There are books and online courses as well as in-person training. You can find out more at https://www.heartmath.org.

Breathing through your nose

Let's start with the basics: nose breathing is one of the few scientifically proven methods for turning off the stress response and turning on the healing 'rest, digest, calm and restore' mode through conscious control. Simply breathing in through the nose rather than the mouth means you are improving your vagal tone, and just five minutes a day can make a significant difference.

- First, find five minutes where you won't be interrupted. As you get better at this you won't need to shut yourself away, but it helps when you're beginning if you can.
- Sit comfortably.
- Close your eyes. Notice how you are naturally breathing and allow your belly to relax so it can expand outwards as you breathe in. As you breathe out your belly will naturally come back in towards your spine. Don't force it.
- Breathe slowly in through your nose and see if you can make a noise like the sea as you take the breath deep into your sinuses. This is known as ujjayi breathing. Release the breath through a slightly opened mouth with a deep, slow sigh. These sounds are helpful as they add to the stimulation of your vagus nerve.
- As this becomes more natural, increase the length of the out breath. It can be helpful to count. Aim to have your out breath twice as long as your in breath.
- Once this is comfortable, hold your in breath for a while before breathing out. Once you have emptied your lungs, hold there again. Work towards a counting pattern of in for 4 – hold for 7 – out for 8 – hold until you feel the natural urge to breathe in again. Repeat this pattern for a few minutes.
- Take time for a few natural breaths before stopping the practice as this allows the body to resume balance and for the vagus nerve to reset. Aim to do this practice twice daily. It works really well on waking and just before you go to sleep.

The basic technique

Developed by Stanley Rosenberg, a physical therapist and vagal nerve specialist, this simple technique is highly effective at triggering rest and restoring vagal activation.

- Sit or lie down comfortably.
- Interlock your fingers and place them behind your head, elbows wide.
- Keep your head in a central position while you take a few deep breaths in and out through the nose.
- Maintaining the central position of your head, move your eyes to try to look at one of your elbows. Keep your eyes looking out to the side for 30–60 seconds. At some point during this time you might spontaneously sigh, yawn or feel some bodily release. That's the vagus nerve activating.
- Repeat on the other side.

Aim to do this every day – it's a great way to help your body prepare for sleep.

Gargling

The vibrational action of gargling helps to activate the vagus nerve where it travels through the sinuses, throat and voice box.

- Gargle for 30 seconds morning and night.
- If you start to produce tears, you know you have done enough.
- If you don't produce tears, keeping practising and eventually you might notice your eyes watering. This is a sign of the vagus nerve kicking into action.

Singing, vigorous humming, omming or chanting

These are all easy ways to kick-start your vagal training for the same reason as gargling. If you are depressed and anxious, you probably don't feel inclined to sing as it's largely a happiness response. As with many of these techniques, you may need to dig deep when you start out doing something you simply don't want to do, but that's when they have the most power.

Put on one of your favourite songs, turn it up loud and sing along with it. If singing isn't your thing, humming is a very powerful alternative, clinically proven to improve your rest-and-digest, parasympathetic response. [80]

Full-body shaking

As with gargling, singing and humming, vagal stimulation can be achieved through vibration. A 60-second full-body shake can be extremely effective as a vagal nerve reset. It's something you'll see in the natural world when an animal has escaped being chased by a predator or a kitten has got scared by falling off the sofa – they'll shake off the adrenaline and discharge the tense energy with a good, full-body, top-to-toe mega-jiggle.

Shaking sends a signal to the limbic centre (emotion regulation) in the brain that the danger has passed, allowing the body to release tension and return to a balanced state. This is important because without the signal that the danger has passed, the state of high alert becomes normalised, making it increasingly difficult for the vagus nerve to kick in. Over time this can lead to biological changes in the brain, where the neurons have fired together so often that they wire together and become fixed in 'stress-on' mode.

Break up this hard-wiring with regular 60-second full-body shakes. You should find you have a lovely sense of tension releasing and a gentle tingle in your fingertips and toes as your body discharges nitric oxide, which lowers blood pressure and heart rate.

Laughing and smiling

It may sound silly, even insensitive, to suggest this to someone who is depressed and barely able to lift their head and look you in the eye, or to someone so anxious they are on the edge of tears. However, forcing a smile, even when you really don't feel like it, is a great way to trick your mind into believing you are feeling better than you actually are, and that in turn changes your biochemistry. This is one of the simplest and quickest ways to begin the process of reducing your stress hormones, lowering your blood pressure and increasing the feel-good brain chemicals. As the facial muscles perform a smile, your amygdala, the area of the brain involved in emotional regulation, releases the neurotransmitters associated with a happy and positive state. Conversely, in a study on over 11,000 people, scowling caused them to feel angrier and frowning made them feel sadder. [81]

No one is suggesting that smiling is a cure for depression or anxiety, but it is worth giving it a try and see if you notice even a tiny lightening of your mood or reduction in stress. If, in the depths of feeling awful, you force your mouth into a smiley shape, especially if you can also bring in some focused nasal breathing (as described earlier), the signals that go to your brain will change. As you engage the muscles that make your face smile or force a belly laugh, the vagus nerve is activated, signalling to your brain that you are experiencing something positive for your well-being. The brain doesn't know the difference between forced and natural contraction of these muscles, so you get the positive outcome even if you're not truly feeling it.

Like so many of these vagal toning tips, this takes time and practice. It is one of the most effective tools at shifting your state to have a different perspective and therefore coping strategy for whatever is taxing you.

Triggering the gag reflex

If you're brave, this is especially powerful to kick-start the vagus nerve. When you're cleaning your teeth or scraping your tongue (a great practice for good oral health that is key for good gut and brain health), put your toothbrush or tongue scraper as far to the back of your tongue as you can and you should find your gag reflex is triggered. The vagus nerve is what causes us to gag, choke or vomit if there's something stuck in our throat or if we've eaten something nasty.

Bilabial trill

Also known as a 'lip trill', this is a great way to get vibration through the vagus nerve. Some people can naturally do this with ease, for others it takes practice.

- Exhale through your mouth with your lips lightly pursed so that your lips vibrate and make a noise like a horse. Try doing this when going about your daily business and keep it going for a few minutes.
- You can also double up a lip trill with humming for added benefit.
- Do this when you notice you are getting irritated, overwhelmed or anxious.
- It's also great to do with children who are struggling with their mood regulation.

Cold water exposure

Cold water is well known as a vagal tonic as it stimulates brain chemicals to calm your breathing and your nervous system. Not only is cold water exposure invigorating, increasing blood and lymph circulation and immune function, it has also been clinically proven to help with depression.

- Start gently by splashing cold water on your face a few times just after you wake up.
- If you're feeling particularly tense or dysregulated you can apply ice cubes to the flat bones behind your ears (mastoid

- bone) or an icepack on your chest.
- The next step is to immerse your face in a bowl of very cold water. Add some ice cubes to cold water to really chill it down. Take a deep breath and put your face in the water while holding your breath. When you feel the need to take a breath, lift your head out, catch your breath and then try again.
- Better still, try to have 15–30 seconds of cold water exposure during or at the end of a shower. The thought of this can be extremely challenging and off-putting, but do give it a go. After 7–10 days of consistent cold water exposure, the body adjusts and the experience gets far easier to tolerate, until it becomes a habit that you then miss if you don't do it. When starting cold showering, try not to immediately tense and hold your breath against the cold. Rather, force yourself to take slow, deep, deliberate breaths, in through the nose with a long exhale out through your mouth. Your sympathetic nervous system will calm down allowing the parasympathetic to take over and you will find you can receive the cold water and feel the benefit rather than fighting the cold. The more you practise this, the more natural it will become and the greater the benefits to your vagal resilience and production of feel-good hormones like endorphins.

GEEK BOX

Cold exposure

Cold exposure activates the cholinergic neurons of the vagal pathway, releasing the neurotransmitter acetylcholine, which tells young lungs to breathe and your nervous system to calm.

If cold showering doesn't do it for you, find out if there is an open water group near you. This is more common than you might realise, with lakes, canals and rivers being used by groups who meet regularly and support each other in this practice. Clinically depressed people have been prescribed cold water swimming as a therapy for drug-resistant depression with amazing results. For safety reasons never go alone unless you are extremely experienced. Having a set time and a group of supportive people to meet with can really help get you into the habit, keep you accountable and provide you with the precious mental health benefits of social interaction.

Positive social connection

Social connection is one of the key factors most commonly identified as necessary to live a long and healthy life. When you are feeling anxious or depressed it can be last thing you feel like doing, but it could be the very thing you need to help change your biochemistry and support your vagal tone. Having a regular group to meet with for some kind of activity, be it knitting, a book group, walking or just a get-together, can be extremely helpful so you don't have to put any additional effort into thinking about what to do, where to go or who you might be meeting. Having a regular group also brings a sense of belonging and community that creates social bonds. This takes us back to the primal days of needing to be part of a tribe for survival. To reinforce this behaviour we make oxytocin, the love and connection hormone.

Regularly being part of a group often results in friendships and a support system so there's someone to notice if you've not been for a while and they can check in with you and make sure you're OK. Local gardening groups, swimming or walking groups are all great, or maybe consider offering a few hours to a local charity or old people's home. If that feels too much, begin simply by imagining what you might like to do. Have a look at what's on offer nearby and keep going back to the idea of starting on something like this until it feels less overwhelming.

Acupuncture and body work

Physical therapy of any form can be transformative. A lot of good research exists on the power of acupuncture for rebalancing nerves and hormones, but any form of body work like massage, shiatsu or reflexology can aid in vagal tone, helping to de-rev the sympathetic nervous system, boosting the rest, relax and recover mode. Some people feel very uncomfortable being touched by someone they don't know, so having a hand or foot massage can be a safe start and is wonderfully therapeutic. Shiatsu is a clothes-on body treatment, so that too can feel easier as a starting point.

Red light therapy

Infrared and near-infrared light therapy is becoming increasingly popular for more than just getting a healthy sweat on, although sweating is excellent for supporting detoxification. The specific frequencies of infrared and near-infrared allow the light waves to penetrate our cells, increasing the rate of energy production due to the activation of the mitochondria, the power providers and communicators within our cells. Traditionally used on inflamed damaged joints and muscles, red light therapy is also being used to help ease pain all around the body and improve sleep, and it may even assist in weight loss. Some research also suggests red light therapy applied to the abdomen can increase gut microbial function and ease gastric issues like IBS and gastritis. Many of these benefits are thought to be due to the red light's positive impact on vagal tone.

Commercial infrared saunas are available at some health clubs and gyms. Home devices in the form of infrared blankets, lamps and panels are becoming more readily available at more reasonable prices. Due to the multiple benefits for physical, metabolic, detox processes and gut health, this might be something you want to investigate.

Sleep

There is an intimate relationship between our sleep pattern and our mental health. Mental and emotional regulation is dependent on good sleep, yet most mental health conditions include disrupted sleep as part of the diagnosis. Insomnia, an extreme and extended period of inability to sleep, is one of the symptoms used to diagnose depressive and anxiety disorders.

Poor sleep includes sleeping too much as well as too little, struggling to get to sleep or waking often through the night. It can be a vicious cycle, with poor sleep contributing to poor mental health and mental health issues disrupting quality sleep. It is no wonder one of the most effective torture techniques is sleep deprivation. The cumulative effects of sleep loss have been associated with a wide range of health problems, including high blood pressure, diabetes, obesity, increased risk of heart attack and stroke and depression, anxiety and addictive behaviours. Matthew Walker, a professor at UC Berkeley and author of Why We Sleep, comments:

> *Just one poor night's sleep results in the deep, emotional centre of the brain to be 60% more reactive, emotional, irrational.* [82]

In a study in conjunction with Harvard Medical School, Walker and his team assigned 26 healthy people to a normal sleep group or a sleep-deprived group. Both groups were shown 100 images that started out neutral but then increased in degree of negativity. The sleep-deprived group showed significantly greater and more intense activation in the brain in response to the disturbing images.

> *'The size of the increase truly surprised us,' Walker said. 'The emotional centers of the brain were over 60% more reactive under conditions of sleep deprivation than in subjects who had obtained a normal night of sleep.'*

Those who were suffering from lack of sleep also showed a stronger connection to the brain's primitive, impulsive regions and less to the rational prefrontal lobe, which normally acts as a check on emotions. Malfunctioning brain circuits between the amygdala and the prefrontal lobe are associated with depression.

> 'This study demonstrates the dangers of not sleeping enough. Sleep deprivation fractures the brain mechanisms that regulate key aspects of our mental health,' Walker said. 'Sleep appears to restore our emotional brain circuits, and in doing so prepares us for the next day's challenges and social interactions.' [83]

If we can sleep well, our ability to cope with the stresses and strains of life measurably improves. Our tolerance for hard challenges and our resolve to look after ourselves better are higher if we've had a restorative night's sleep. If you are someone who doesn't sleep well, this can feel like a failure and drive more anxiety, but don't be disheartened. There is so much you can do to improve your sleep hygiene, setting your body and brain up with the right cues at the right time to get a good night's sleep.

Wilderness guides include the 'rule of 3', meaning we can live without oxygen for 3 minutes, without water for 3 days and without food for 3 weeks. Yet only 7 days of little to no sleep can have serious and lasting mental and physical health consequences.

Phases of sleep

During sleep we go through cycles of light, deep and REM (rapid eye movement) sleep. Different jobs get done around the body and brain during these phases:

- Light sleep (50–60% of our total sleep time) includes some repair and cleaning as well as memory consolidation and we even improve the coordination of our muscles. Just because it's termed light, since it's when we're easily woken, doesn't mean it's not important.

- Deep sleep tends to follow light sleep. This is where the brain waves slow right down, heart rate and blood pressure are at their lowest and the brain goes into deep repair mode. The organs and tissues around the body are cleansed and restored while the microglial cells that coat the neurons in the brain kick into gear to clear out any build-up of plaques and toxins. This process is critical for the management of inflammation in the brain.
- REM sleep is our dream sleep. It's where we experience emotional regulation, process information that we've been exposed to during the day and continue with the cleaning and repair processes. Ideally, our deep and REM sleep combined should be around 50% of our total sleep.

Programming sleep

For us to sleep well, certain signals need to be in play throughout the day. Sleep drive is the term used for all the factors that contribute to getting a good night's sleep. As the science of sleep has advanced over recent years, one of the most important findings for a strong sleep drive is what you do when you get up, a whole 16 hours or so before you're next going to be asleep.

Natural light exposure in the early morning

Bright morning light suppresses melatonin and adenosine, the sleep chemicals, and triggers cortisol, the get-up-and-go hormone. This activates the circadian clock inside our eye, brain and skin cells, which signal the awake response while also programming a sleep response 16 hours later, when the brain will produce the sleep chemicals again. Don't expect to fix your sleep issues by desperately trying to turn off at bedtime. Set your own body clock with morning light as soon after getting up as possible and your body will naturally know when to turn off at night.

Even on cloudy, dull days, it's worth getting outside for 10–15 minutes and looking up at the sky with naked eyes (no sunglasses, although don't look directly at the sun). Try to do this while the sun is still coming up. On bright sunny days just 5 minutes of being outside should be enough. If you can't get outside, sit by a window where the morning sunlight is coming in.

Daylight exposure at sunset

Somewhat less potent but still useful is to get some natural daylight exposure when the sun is setting. The setting sun gives off a different spectrum of light, opposite to that of the rising morning sun. The eyes receive this information and tell the brain that the sun is going down and that it's time to suppress the awake hormones and begin to release the sleep chemicals.

If you've ever watched the sunset on the horizon, you might have experienced the calm and soothing effect this has on your mood and state of being. Of course, most of us most of the time can't do this, but at least try to catch a glimpse of the sun going down in the late afternoon or evening to help your sleep clock kick in on time.

Block blue light at night

Blue light doesn't look blue, it's a hidden spectrum of light coming off our various devices. Screens including HDTV, smartphones and computers give off blue light, which is the same spectrum as when the sun is high in the sky in the middle of the day. Therefore, if your eyes are seeing blue light in the evening from your screens, the brain interprets this as the sun still being high and that can lead to a delay in or suppression of the release of your sleep chemicals.

Some people are far more sensitive to blue light than others. If you aren't sleeping well, especially if you're unable to get off to sleep, it's worth experimenting with blue light blocking apps or blue light blocking glasses and getting good about not looking at screens, especially if you don't have blocking tools, at least an hour before you want to be asleep. Additionally, get into the habit of turning off some of the lights in the house to create a dimmer environment. Household lights, especially LED ceiling lights, can also trigger the awake cycle, so where possible use low-level lamps and dim ceiling lights if possible.

> *Evidence suggests that people who are regularly exposed to long periods of artificial light exposure at night and have reduced exposure to natural daylight have an increased risk of depression.* [84]

Wake and sleep times

Your body, including your gut microbes, your liver and your brain, has different modes of function at different times of the day. It likes to know when to do what. If you go to bed and get up at roughly the same time consistently, your body will much more readily and fully switch into sleep mode or awake mode. This is one of the main reasons jetlag can be so disorientating. Your body wants to do its night-time and daytime jobs at the time it's used to and having a time zone change disrupts that, causing all sorts of digestive and sleep issues.

Consistency in this area can be especially challenging for people with depression who are prone to oversleeping. Being disciplined about getting up, even if you cannot bear to face the day, can be an important step to a happier brain. Having a bedtime and a getting-up time that you aim to hit within a 30-minute range on a daily basis can make all the difference to your mental and physical well-being.

Magnesium

As discussed in Chapter Eight, a magnesium glycinate supplement is a great sleep aid. Having a bath with two good handfuls of Epsom salts (magnesium sulphate) is also a safe, well-studied sleep intervention. Magnesium is very relaxing, so dosing up with it prior to bedtime helps the vagus nerve switch your system into sleep, rest and repair mode, while also aiding in muscle relaxation and the release of physical tension.

This is especially useful for people who get muscle cramps at night or restless leg syndrome. An Epsom salt bath allows the magnesium to enter the body transdermally, through the skin, and the magnesium glycinate supplement helps calm the brain and body as both the glycine and the magnesium aid in regulation of the nervous system. It's best not to have both a bath and a magnesium supplement together, as this can cause a very rapid blood pressure drop in some people.

Body temperature

Deep sleep is restorative for our mental well-being, but is often the most elusive of the sleep phases. Keeping cool at night is really important, as we don't enter deep sleep unless our body temperature drops slightly.

- Aim to keep your bedroom at or below 18 °C/65 °F.
- Have a window open if this is an option.
- Wear light, natural bedclothes to allow your body temperature to naturally drop when you are asleep.
- Set your heating to go off at night.
- If you sleep next to someone who gets very hot, consider separate duvets or bedclothes so you can adjust accordingly.

Sleep disruptors

Some common lifestyle factors are major suppressors to the production of natural sleep hormones and sleep signals, so think about how you can avoid their detrimental effects:

- Caffeine blocks the sleep chemical adenosine from building up throughout the day, which weakens your drive to sleep.

Around half the caffeine stays active for up to 8 hours after consumption and a quarter is still active for up to 12 hours. Everyone clears caffeine at different rates. If you are not sleeping well, it is worth stopping any caffeine-containing drinks (coffee, tea, including green tea, and energy drinks) by midday at the latest, ideally earlier.

- Alcohol is another major sleep disruptor. It can be relaxing – it's actually a sedative – but it creates heat, preventing deep-cycle sleep, and often causes gut microbial disturbance. Alcohol inhibits fat burning at night, when we depend on fat stores for fuel, and the effects on the brain can be depressive.
- Eating late is a huge sleep disruptor. Wherever possible leave at least three hours from finishing eating to bedtime. If that isn't possible have something light to eat, as a heavy meal close to bedtime will negatively affect both sleep and digestion, leaving you prone to acid reflux, bloating and being hot and restless throughout the night.
- Exercising late is not suitable for most people. Exercise heats us up and raises stress hormones, both a problem for a good night's sleep.
- Watching the news or anything too aggravating, stimulating or challenging can trigger the stress hormones to rise when they should be reducing. Wherever possible don't check emails or work on something taxing before bed – it's just too wiring for what should be a time for calming down.

Moving your body

There are many reasons why moving your body more is a good idea. Most of us know that exercise is good for heart health, weight management, diabetes and vascular health. All of these relate to metabolic well-being. As mental health is now being looked at, at least in part, as a metabolic condition of the brain, it's no wonder that exercise benefits the production of brain energy too. Better energy leads to better functioning of all our bodily systems. Georgia Ede, a

Harvard-trained psychiatrist specialising in nutrition science, emphasises:

> 'If you improve metabolic health, mental health tends to follow.' [85]

Many scientific studies have conclusively shown that exercise changes the way the brain works in remarkable ways, having a greater impact on mood and neurochemical balance than anything pharmacological. A meta-analysis (a review of lots of studies done on the same subject) combining findings on nearly 200,000 people with depression concluded:

> *This systematic review and meta-analysis of associations between physical activity and depression suggests significant mental health benefits from being physically active, even at levels below the public health recommendations. Health practitioners should therefore encourage any increase in physical activity to improve mental health.* [86]

There has been a lot of research over the last decade looking at exercise and mental health and one of the main benefits appears to be the increase in blood to the brain. Around a litre of blood is passing through the brain every minute. Exercising increases this blood flow, delivering more oxygen and vital nutrients, allowing the brain to be better fuelled. Clearance of the toxins constantly being produced by the brain via the lymphatic system is also greatly enhanced through physical movement. This increase in blood flow appears to create better communication between the different regions of the brain too.

As with diabetes of the body, diabetes or poor glucose regulation in the brain improves with exercise. Exercise also positively affects the gut microbes, including the diversity of the happy gut bugs; in particular the gut microbes that increase with exercise tend to be the ones that produce short-chain fatty acids, [87] those compounds like butyrate that are directly associated with a healthier gut and a happier brain. As exercise improves the gut microbes, not only does their communication with the brain get better, so too does the condition of the gut lining. A healthy gut lining greatly reduces the chances of inflammatory compounds leaking out of the gut and passing into the brain, critical in the management of good mental health.

> *Resistance exercise training significantly reduced depressive symptoms among adults regardless of health status ... frequency or improvements in strength.* [88]

The function of our mitochondria also greatly improves with exercise. Mitochondria create the energy and intelligence of our cells. The more energy the mitochondria make, the more the body and brain can thrive. The good gut microbes and mitochondria are both hugely correlated with better mental health status.

Some studies have looked at how when we exercise muscles use up certain chemicals that, if allowed to build up and circulate around the brain, could cause a toxic build-up that is associated with depression. Conversely, when we move our muscles, they produce chemicals that have been termed 'hope molecules' because they improve resilience to stress and symptoms of depression.[89] Exercise is also key for maintaining the function of tiny blood vessels in the brain that transport our brain chemicals. Regular exercise helps to keep these tiny vessels open and can even promote the growth of new blood vessels in the brain. [90]

Exercise may feel like the very last thing you can face doing, so start gently and think about being more active as opposed to having to do lots of structured exercise. Taking a short walk, ideally outdoors, gently swinging your arms and pushing your pace just a little faster than your normal walking speed, can bring significant and lasting benefit. As this becomes more comfortable, try to get out for a walk every day or every other day. Eventually start to pick up your pace and walk a little further. Having a walking buddy can be lovely. Find someone with whom you can be yourself, where if you don't feel like chatting you can comfortably walk in silence. It's helpful if this is someone who doesn't expect you to 'put on a brave face' or cheer up. Make sure you have someone whose company you welcome, who brings comfort and support in a non-demanding way, yet who keeps you accountable to getting out for your walk on a regular basis.

Any form of exercise is good: aerobic or resistance, long or short. Moving your body, making your muscles work, your heart pump and your lungs increase their uptake of oxygen, is what is important. The best form of exercise is the one that you will do most readily.

> *Exercise is more effective than medicines to manage mental health.* [91]

Light exposure

As well as helping with our sleep drive, getting regular doses of daylight has been shown to help with mood regulation and depression. Sunlight improves our mood in many ways, by increasing levels of vitamin D, a key mood-regulating vitamin, but also by stimulating our vagus nerve. Sun exposure increases the production of a set of hormones known collectively as melanocyte-stimulating hormone (MSH). UVB rays from the sun increase the number of MSH receptors in the body, which then allows more MSH to be used and this helps keep our vagal tone in check. No wonder it feels so good to get some sunshine on our skin.

If getting outdoors is too hard due to your physical or mental health circumstances, sitting in front of a light box is a great alternative. Light boxes give off a specific spectrum of light shown to have a direct anti-depressant effect. These are used widely for people with seasonal affective disorder, who suffer greatly with low mood and energy during the dark months of the year, but other forms of depression have been shown to benefit from 30-minute morning exposure to a full-spectrum light box. This appears to work thanks to the stimulation of the mood-regulation regions of the brain.

Mindfulness

Slowing down a busy mind or breaking the cycle of negative self-talk can be very challenging. A meditation or mindfulness practice offers structure to something that might otherwise feel elusive and frustrating. Studies show that mindfulness reduces inflammation and oxidative stress, providing a more healing and balanced environment in the body and allowing your energy-providing mitochondria to feel safe enough to power up your cells. Yoga, mindfulness and meditation classes are being recommended by various bodies within the NHS to improve outcomes of mood disorders, cancer treatment and high blood pressure.

When life is already a struggle, being still and sitting with your thoughts can feel unbearable. Some people find their anxiety worsens when they try to sit in a calm and reflective way. This is entirely understandable. Being distracted with the TV, snacking or generally keeping busy can feel far preferable to looking inwards. However, many studies show that learning to look internally, trying to be present rather than thinking about what has happened or might happen, is an important tool for robust mental health.

With a wide range of smartphone apps, YouTube videos and books available as a guide, learning a structured 10–20-minute practice where your breathing is regulated and your focus is on being present, letting thoughts pass without judgement, can be transformative over time. Guided meditations can help with the mental chatter that can feel disruptive, while other people find music or a voice too distracting. Various wearable tech devices are available to help with regulating breathing patterns and improving vagal tone for those who find mindful practices hard, while for others being calm and quiet, just giving oneself permission to stop, can bring surprising benefits.

Walking in silence can be a mindful and restorative practice where you observe your surroundings and watch for the distracting thoughts that take you out of the moment. This can be achieved even in a busy city or on a bustling town high street. However, most people will gain more benefit by walking in nature where possible.

Journaling

If you find mindful, calm, meditative-type practices just too challenging, a helpful alternative is to write down your thoughts and feelings. Allow a free flow of words without censorship or trying to make sense of what you are writing. Many people find that once they start journaling, they experience a great sense of calm.

When we are thinking about things, multiple thoughts can get jumbled up together, creating lots of noise with little resolution. When we are writing or speaking out loud, our thoughts have to go through a different processing system in the brain to become more coherent, and in so doing we can find resolution or at least a different understanding of the thoughts and feelings that are otherwise intrusive and seemingly unresolvable.

Some people find journaling first thing in the morning a useful time to clear some mental baggage before the day begins. Others prefer a night-time mental unloading to help them sleep. If you can, buy a lovely notebook to use to make the process have extra meaning and value. You may never go back and look at what you've written, and that's fine. It's not a diary as such, it's moving information to a safe storage space to free up your mind. There are no rules, no right or wrong, just be as free as you can be.

Gratitude

Gratitude and compassion are two very strong senses that promote improvements in vagal tone and an increase in gut–brain axis communication and brain chemical regulation. Gratitude inhibits fear and anxiety, reduces stress hormones and improves sleep quality. Therefore, getting into the practice of being more grateful can be very therapeutic. Elite athletes, business moguls and Buddhist monks promote the practice of gratitude to improve mental, physical and spiritual well-being.

A gratitude practice might sound unrealistic in light of your struggles. However, taking a few moments every day to write a list (which could be part of your journaling) of anything you can think of that gives you a sense of gratitude can be deeply therapeutic. From having a bed to lie in to water coming out of the tap, from having enough food to eat to having meaningful relationships and everything in between, even in the most desperate of situations there is usually something we can be grateful for.

Essential oils

Extracted and concentrated plant oils can have offer immediate relief of symptoms for some people. Not to be underestimated, the beautiful scents don't not just provide pleasure, these potent volatile oils have many therapeutic effects. Aromatherapy practitioners are expert in this field, carefully combining different oils to create bespoke blends based on need.

Essential oils are a beneficial alternative to air-freshening sprays, plug-ins and scented candles. Most 'air-freshening' products give off nasty compounds that you are breathing in. Some people are unknowingly highly sensitive to these man-made chemicals that are known to have endocrine (hormone) and neurologically disruptive effects.

There are a few essential oils that can be safely used on a daily basis without expert advice, inhaled deeply through the nose or sprinkled on clothing or bedding. Go by how you immediately respond to the smell – is it uplifting and pleasant or off-putting? Trust your instincts and use the oils that suit you.

- Lavender is known to have a profound calming effect on the nervous system. It can be inhaled or used on clothing or directly on the skin. It helps ease tension, reduce blood pressure and calm nerves. It's lovely to sprinkle on your bedclothes at night.
- Roman chamomile is another soothing oil that helps with sleep and calming the mind.

- Valerian is mildly sedative so is great for sleep and relaxation.
- Rosemary has anti-depressant properties and helps with memory recall and general brain activity.
- Bergamot, from the citrus family, is wonderfully uplifting. It is great to use early in the day to give you a boost. Combined with lime essential oil, the blend has wonderful calming and uplifting properties, great for anxiety and feeling panicked.
- Patchouli is commonly used in incense and is often associated with yogic and meditative practices. It has been shown to help with stress and depression.

Conclusion

As the field of psychiatry grapples with the uncomfortable truth that the treatment options used for depression and anxiety are outdated, often ineffective, with challenging side effects and that they do not address the underlying causes of mental ill-health, more and more patients and practitioners are choosing to address mental health problems with a whole-body approach. For many, it's working in incredible ways.

With or without psychiatric medication, a body that is metabolically well is, by definition, going to manage mental health better than one whose internal systems are struggling to create and maintain balance. The whole-body approach is complex, nuanced and individual, requiring far greater dedication than popping a pill, but it does offer the potential for lasting change without any negative side effects. Often a situation needs to get very bad before there is enough impetus for change to happen. You can choose to circumvent this process and take charge of your life now. With a little focus and fortitude along with a good dose of curiosity and self-care, you can start to find ways out of bad habits and create new, healthier relationships to food and lifestyle choices.

I have seen clinically, and experienced personally, the staggering, often rapid gains that can be made by a change in diet and lifestyle. I am confident in my belief that helping your body to work better will help your brain, whatever the underlying cause of your mental ill-health. Think about which aspect of your lifestyle are not supporting your health – is it not enough sleep, sitting too much, eating fast food too often, using alcohol to numb your pain? Make one change, just one shift in a new direction, and that will lead to the next and then the next small change that allows healing to happen, nudging the body towards a happier mode of function and more tolerance for stress and emotional pain.

I don't underestimate for one moment how daunting this change of approach might feel. Even thinking about where to begin might be exhausting or anxiety provoking. So start small, be gentle with yourself and trust that your body has a wisdom that will support your efforts given the smallest of opportunities. For the many mental health sufferers who have already chosen to tackle their whole-body wellness head on, change is happening surprisingly quickly, and each change drives their motivation and commitment to continue because the rewards greatly outweigh the effort involved.

> *'Metabolism is not easy or simple, but it IS the only way to understand mental disorders.'*
> Chris Palmer MD, author of Brain Energy

Remember, your body is constantly receiving and interpreting the information that's coming into it: whether you're smiling or frowning; whether you're eating foods that heal or harm your gut microbes; the quality of your thoughts and self-talk; how much sleep you're getting and its quality. Everything you do, think and feel is resonating through your gut microbiome and up to your brain. Your brain takes that information and makes sense of it. What you do and how you live drive how you feel, which drives how you think and behave.

The information you input daily through your lifestyle choices becomes your mental health experience.

If you have an unhappy brain, change the information you are sending to it. This starts by healing more and harming less those incredible, non-human inhabitants of your digestive system, the gut microbes. It is a hard reality that for many of us modern life is challenging our equilibrium, driving up inflammation, driving down gut–brain communication and leaving us under-nourished and over-stressed in the process. If you start to notice, care about and take action to nurture your gut microbes, they will pay you back in ways that we still don't fully understand, but that we do know can help to heal an unhappy brain.

I hope this book has provided you with at least an inkling of what is possible for you. Take that first step – use this book as a starting point for making changes in how you nourish your body and mind to enable a happier brain. Decide to prioritise yourself and your whole body's well-being. Be patient, be gentle and be aware of what is changing within you day by day, sleep by sleep, step by step.

I wish you well on your health journey to a happier brain.

Appendix

Recommended foods list

These foods are all gut and brain friendly. Aim to include 10 of these foods daily or 30 weekly – the wider the variety the better. Not everyone will like all of these foods, but be brave and try those you're not familiar with. Aim for these foods to make up at least 80% of your diet.

Truly super superfoods

- Fermented foods (see below)
- Green tea
- Bone broth (cooked for at least 12 hours)
- Ginger and turmeric
- Raw cacao
- Garlic and onions
- Cruciferous vegetables (see below)
- Bitter-tasting leaves
- Fresh herbs

Fermented foods

- Vegetable ferments: sauerkraut, kimchi
- Dairy ferments: live, natural yogurt, dairy (or coconut) kefir
- Soy ferments: miso, tempeh, tamari soy sauce, natto

- Raw apple cider vinegar
- Kombucha and water kefir drinks (they should not be sweet)

Best animal products

- Cold water, wild oily fish
- Raw, full-fat milk, cream and unpasteurised cheeses, especially those made of milk from goats, sheep or brown cows
- Pasture-fed, outdoor-reared meats and wild game

Best fats and oils

- Extra virgin coconut oil – good for high-heat cooking
- Extra virgin olive oil – use liberally but not for high-heat cooking
- Butter and ghee from organic, grass-fed animals
- Good-quality (from free-range animals) lard, goose fat and duck fat
- Avocado oil

Best fruits

- Berries – especially blueberries, blackberries, redcurrants, blackcurrants, strawberries and raspberries, in season or British frozen
- Citrus fruits
- Green, sour apples, especially Bramley apples stewed with their skins on
- Kiwi fruit – wash well and eat the skin
- Stone fruits (in season) – apricots, cherries, plums
- Green or very pale yellow bananas (1/3 is a portion), which are full of resistant starch

Best vegetables

- Alliums – leeks, garlic, onions (especially red onions), spring onions and chives
- Brassicas – broccoli and broccoli sprouts, cabbage, cauliflower, Brussel sprouts, kale, rocket, spring greens
- Brightly coloured vegetables – peppers, squashes, tomatoes, spinach, chard, kohlrabi, watercress
- Bitter leaves – radicchio, chicory, root of Romaine and sweet gem lettuce

Best whole grains

- A maximum of 25% of the total meal and ideally soaked overnight in water with a little vinegar:
- Wholegrain rye bread, especially sourdough rye (not if avoiding gluten)
- Quinoa, a pseudo-grain
- Amaranth, a pseudo-grain
- Buckwheat groats, a pseudo-grain (or 100% buckwheat soba noodles)
- Millet
- Whole (jumbo) organic oats, in moderation
- Pot barley (not if avoiding gluten)

Best pulses

- Dried beans, peas etc. need to be soaked for at least 24 hours, then cook them at a rolling boil for at least 20 minutes and replace the water, bring to a boil and simmer until very soft.
- All lentils
- Any beans or pulses in water – tinned or in jars
- 'ZenB' pasta or other pulse-based pastas

Best nuts and seeds

Soak nuts and seeds for improved digestion and nutrition. Smell nuts, especially walnuts, and if they smell rancid do not eat them. Keep all nuts and seeds in a cool, dark place. Always soak chia and flax seeds.

- Chia and flax seeds
- Pumpkin and sunflower seeds
- Walnuts
- Pecans
- Macadamia nuts
- Almonds
- Brazil nuts
- Hazelnuts

'Better than most' sweeteners

- Good-quality honey or maple syrup – in very small amounts
- Xylitol
- Allulose

Resources

Fabulous cookbooks for a happy brain

Happy Gut, Happy Mind: How to Feel Good from Within, Eva Kalinik, Piatkus
The Low Carb Italian Kitchen: Modern Mediterranean Recipes for Weight Loss and Good Health, Katie & Giancarlo Caldesi, Kyle Books
Genius Kitchen: Over 100 Easy and Delicious Recipes to Make Your Brain Sharp, Body Strong, and Taste Buds Happy, Max Lugavere, Harper
Ketogenic Global Kitchen: The World's Most Delicious Foods Made Keto & Easy, Elizabeth Jane, Progressive Publishing
The Clever Guts Diet Recipe Book: 150 Delicious Recipes to Mend Your Gut and Boost Your Health and Wellbeing, Clare Bailey, Short Books
Low Carb Cookbook with 4 Ingredients, Pascale Naessens, Lannoo Publishers
The Keto Cure: A New Life in 14 Days, Pascale Naessens, Lannoo Publishers
Unprocess Your Life: The new cookbook to help you break free from ultra-processed foods by Rob Hobson, Thorsons

Healthy eating information

- **Freshwell:** Sensible, practical advice on healthy eating and navigating a low carb way of life
  https://lowcarbfreshwell.com
- **Public Health Collaboration:** A wonderful charity providing valuable free information
  https://phcuk.org

- **Food for the Brain Foundation:** A charity dedicated to informing and supporting those with brain health concerns
  https://foodforthebrain.org

Sites to find registered nutrition experts

- **BANT – British Association for Nutrition and Lifestyle Medicine:** A great resource to find highly qualified nutritional therapists, with a search tool for experts in your area
  https://bant.org.uk
- **Nutritionist Resource:** A search tool to find a specialist nutritionist in your area
  https://www.nutritionist-resource.org.uk
- **IFM – Institute for Functional Medicine:** Medical doctors and other health professionals who have undertaken functional medicine training, which supports the philosophy of whole-body health
  https://www.ifm.org

Suppliers

These are companies I use regularly. I am recommending them purely to offer you an easier and reliable way to source great-quality products, and I do not have any financial or business interest in any of them.

- **Abel & Cole:** Delivery of reliably high-quality organic vegetables, meat, dairy, etc.
  www.abelandcole.co.uk
- **BuyWholefoodsOnline:** A great resource for dried goods like nuts, seeds, pseudo-grains, coconut products including toasted flakes, high-quality coconut oil and tinned coconut milk, raw apple cider vinegar, raw sauerkraut, pulses, etc. A family-run business (nothing to do with a high street health

food chain). www.buywholefoodsonline.co.uk
- **Cytoplan:** A science-based supplement company supplying high-quality, food-based supplements to healthcare professionals and their patients, including a prebiotic powder that I helped develop (PreBio Restore) to easily increase levels of highly effective probiotic fibres in the diet. To find a practitioner that can advise you on Cytoplan products, contact the company directly or use the sites listed above to find a registered nutritional therapist.
www.cytoplan.co.uk
- **Agua de Madre:** For really tasty, authentically made water kefir (fermented water containing live microbes). A great, healthy alternative to alcohol and mixers. They also have kits to make water kefir at home.
Agua de Madre https://aguademadre.co.uk/
- **Happy Kombucha:** Supplier of live cultures for making dairy kefir.
www.happykombucha.com
- **My New Roots:** A blog for great healthy recipes, including Life-Changing Bread and Life-Changing Crackers, which are gluten-free, high-soluble-fibre, tasty alternatives.
www.mynewroots.org
- **Symprove:** Manufacturer and supplier of a liquid probiotic for a gentle top-up of happy gut microbes, proven to help with constipation and to have an anti-inflammatory effect on the gut and brain.
www.symprove.com

Notes

[1] Dr Georgia Ede, Harvard-trained psychiatrist on Bipolarcast. Ep15. October 2022: https://www.youtube.com/watch?v=fyWfFHnIUIY

[2] https://foodandmoodcentre.com.au/2016/07/diet-and-mental-health-in-children-and-adolescents/

[3] Halverson, T., & Alagiakrishnan, K. (2020). Gut microbes in neurocognitive and mental health disorders. Annals of Medicine 52(8)L 423–443. https://doi.org/10.1080/07853890.2020.1808239.

[4] 'The Prophet' by Kahlil Gibram (1923)

[5] https://www.sciencedirect.com/science/article/pii/S0924977X19317237

[6] Rucklidge, J., Johnstone, J., Harrison, R. & Boggis, A. (2011) Micronutrients reduce stress and anxiety in adults with Attention-Deficit/Hyperactivity Disorder following a 7.1 earthquake. *Psychiatry Research* 189(2): 281–287. https://doi.org/10.1016/j.psychres.2011.06.016.

[7] https://www.biomolther.org/journal/view.html?uid=1100&vmd=Full

[8] https://www.ewg.org/sites/default/files/2022-05/EWG_EMF-05.22_C01.pdf

[9] https://www.ncbi.nlm.nih.gov/pmc/articles/PMC8415840/

[10] Natalie Goldberg (2011) *Wild Mind: Living the Writer's Life*, Open Road Media, p. 206.

[11] What causes depression? Harvard Health Publishing, 10 January 2022. www.health.harvard.edu/mind-and-mood/what-causes-depression.

[12] Schroder, H.S., Devendorf, A.., & Zikmund-Fisher, B.J. (2023) Framing depression as a functional signal, not a disease: Rationale and initial randomized controlled trial. Social Science & Medicine 328: 115995. https://doi.org/10.1016/j.socscimed.2023.115995.

[13] Ecks, S. (2021) Depression, deprivation, and dysbiosis: Polyiatrogenesis in multiple chronic illnesses. Culture, Medicine, and Psychiatry 45: 507–524. https://doi.org/10.1007/s11013-020-09699-x.

[14] Tian, Y.E., Di Biase, M.A., Mosley, P.E. et al. (2023) Evaluation of brain-body health in individuals with common neuropsychiatric disorders. JAMA Psychiatry 80(6): 567–576. https://doi.org/10.1001/jamapsychiatry.2023.0791.

[15] Laudisio, A., Antonelli Incalzi, R., Gemma, A. et al. (2018) Use of proton-pump inhibitors is associated with depression: A population-based study. International Psychogeriatrics 30(1): 153–159. https://doi.org/ 10.1017/S1041610217001715.

[16] https://www.sciencedirect.com/science/article/abs/pii/S1751499111000060

[17] Joana Araújo, J., Cai, J., and Stevens, J. (2019) Prevalence of optimal metabolic health in American adults: National Health and Nutrition Examination Survey 2009–2016. Metabolic Syndrome and Related Disorders 17(1). https://doi.org/10.1089/met.2018.0105.

[18] Goldman, B. (2021) Insulin resistance doubles risk of major depressive disorder, Stanford study finds. Stanford Medicine, 22 September. https://med.stanford.edu/news/all-news/2021/09/insulin-resistance-major-depressive-disorder.html

[19] Dr Chris Palmer, @ChrisPalmerMD Twitter / X.

[20] https://www.ncbi.nlm.nih.gov/pmc/articles/PMC6361831/

[21] https://www.frontiersin.org/journals/psychiatry/articles/10.3389/fpsyt.2022.951376/full

[22] Adams, R.N., Athinarayanan, S.J., McKenzie, A.L. et al. (2022) Depressive symptoms improve over 2 years of type 2 diabetes treatment via a digital continuous remote care intervention focused on carbohydrate restriction. Journal of Behavioral Medicine 45: 416–427. https://doi.org/10.1007/s10865-021-00272-4.

[23] Sethi, S., Wakeham, D., Ketter., T. et al. (2024) Ketogenic diet intervention on metabolic and psychiatric health in bipolar and schizophrenia: A pilot trial. Psychiatry Research 335: 115866. https://doi.org/10.1016/j.psychres.2024.115866.

[24] Frank, P., Jokela, M., Batty, G.D. et al. (2021) Association between systemic inflammation and individual symptoms of depression: A pooled analysis of 15

population-based cohort studies. *American Journal of Psychiatry* 178(1): 1107–1118. https://doi.org/10.1176/appi.ajp.2021.20121776.

[25] Sima, R. (2023) How inflammation in the body may explain depression in the brain. Washington Post, 23 February. https://www.washingtonpost.com/wellness/2023/02/23/depression-brain-inflammation-treatment.

[26] https://www.frontiersin.org/articles/10.3389/fmed.2022.813204/full

[27] Patel. S., Keating, B.A., & Dale, R.C. (2023) Anti-inflammatory properties of commonly used psychiatric drugs. *Frontiers in Neuroscience* 16. https://doi.org/10.3389/fnins.2022.1039379.

[28] https://www.ncbi.nlm.nih.gov/pmc/articles/PMC5093181/

[29] https://pubmed.ncbi.nlm.nih.gov/22968153/

[30] Ziad, A.T., Abdulmohsen, A.A., Nedal,S.B., & Abderrahman, O. (2023) Brain-inhabiting bacteria and neurodegenerative diseases: The 'brain microbiome' theory. *Frontiers in Aging Neuroscience* 15. https://doi.org/10.3389/fnagi.2023.1240945.

[31] Allouche, H. (2022) Digestive disorders and mental health. News-Medical.net. https://www.news-medical.net/health/Digestive-Disorders-and-Mental-Health.aspx.

[32] Halverson, T., & Alagiakrishnan, K. (2020) Gut microbes in neurocognitive and mental health disorders. *Annals of Medicine* 52(8): 423–443. https://doi.org/10.1080/07853890.2020.1808239.

[33] Varesi, A., Campagnoli, L.I.M., Chirumbolo, S. et al. (2023) The brain-gut-microbiota interplay in depression: A key to design innovative therapeutic approaches. *Pharmacological Research* 192: 106799. https://doi.org/10.1016/j.phrs.2023.106799.

[34] Abautret-Daly, Á., Dempsey, E., Parra-Blanco A. et al. (2018) Gut–brain actions underlying comorbid anxiety and depression associated with inflammatory bowel disease. *Acta Neuropsychiatrica* 30(5): 275–296. https://doi.org/10.1017/neu.2017.3.

[35] The brain-gut connection. John Hopkins Medicine. https://www.hopkinsmedicine.org/health/wellness-and-prevention/the-brain-gut-connection.

[36] Malhi, G.S.,, Bell, E., Bassett, D. et al. (2021) The 2020 Royal Australian and New Zealand College of Psychiatrists clinical practice guidelines for mood

disorders. *Australian & New Zealand Journal of Psychiatry* 55(1): 7–117. https://doi.org/10.1177/0004867420979353.

[37] Sethi, S., Wakeham, D., Ketter, T. et al. (2024) Ketogenic diet intervention on metabolic and psychiatric health in bipolar and schizophrenia: A pilot trial. *Psychiatry Research* 335: 115866. https://doi.org/10.1016/j.psychres.2024.115866.

[38] Lee, Y.Y., Erdogan, A., & Rao, S.S. (2014) How to assess regional and whole gut transit time with wireless motility capsule. *Journal of Neurogastroenterological Motility* 20(2): 265–270. https://doi.org/10.5056/jnm.2014.20.2.265.

[39] Hertzler, S.R., & Clancy, S.M. (2003) Kefir improves lactose digestion and tolerance in adults with lactose maldigestion. *Journal of the American Dietetic Association* 103(5): 582–587. https://doi.org/10.1053/jada.2003.50111.

[40] Siciliano, R.A., Reale, A., Mazzeo, M.F. et al. (2021) Paraprobiotics: A new perspective for functional foods and nutraceuticals. *Nutrients* 13(4): 1225. https://doi.org/10.3390/nu13041225.

[41] KetoFLEX 12/3. Apollo Health. https://www.apollohealthco.com/ketoflex-12-3.

[42] Liu, J., Fang, Y., Cui, L. et al. (2022) Butyrate emerges as a crucial effector of Zhi-Zi-Chi decoctions to ameliorate depression via multiple pathways of brain-gut axis. *Biomedicine & Pharmacotherapy* 149: 112861. https://doi.org/10.1016/j.biopha.2022.112861.

[43] Wapner, J. (2023) The link between our food, gut microbiome and depression. *Washington Post*, 31 January. https://www.washingtonpost.com/wellness/2023/01/31/gut-microbiome-anxiety-depression.

[44] https://www.sciencedirect.com/science/article/abs/pii/S0261561408002227

[45] https://www.sciencedirect.com/science/article/pii/S216183132200833X

[46] https://www.ncbi.nlm.nih.gov/pmc/articles/PMC9730524/

[47] https://pubmed.ncbi.nlm.nih.gov/36555149/

[48] https://www.nature.com/scitable/knowledge/library/evidence-for-meat-eating-by-early-humans-103874273/

[49] Sahih Bukhari 7:71:592.

[50] Bin Sayeed, M.S., Shams, T., Fahim Hossain, S. et al. (2014) Nigella sativa L. seeds modulate mood, anxiety and cognition in healthy adolescent males. *Journal of Ethnopharmacology* 152(1): 156–162. https://doi.org/10.1016/j.

jep.2013.12.050.

[51] Zadeh, A.R., Eghbal, A.F., Mirghazanfari, S.M. et al. (2022) *Nigella sativa* extract in the treatment of depression and serum Brain-Derived Neurotrophic Factor (BDNF) levels. *Journal of Research in Medical Sciences* 27: 28. https://doi.org/10.4103/jrms.jrms_823_21.

[52] https://www.jamesgreenblattmd.com/

[53] https://pubmed.ncbi.nlm.nih.gov/27215959/

[54] Mocking, R.J., Harmsen, I., Assies, J. et al. (2016) Meta-analysis and meta-regression of omega-3 polyunsaturated fatty acid supplementation for major depressive disorder. *Translational Psychiatry* 6(3): e756. https://doi.org/10.1038/tp.2016.29.

[55] Debras, C., Chazelas, E., Sellem, L. et al. (2022) Artificial sweeteners and risk of cardiovascular diseases: Results from the prospective NutriNet-Santé cohort. *BMJ* 378: e071204. https://doi.org/10.1136/bmj-2022-071204.

[56] Higher risk of diabetes with diet drinks. *Diabetes in Control*, 15 February 2013. https://www.diabetesincontrol.com/higher-risk-of-diabetes-with-diet-drinks.

[57] https://www.mdpi.com/1422-0067/22/18/9863

[58] Kimball, S.M., Mirhosseini, N., & Rucklidge, J. (2018) Database analysis of depression and anxiety in a community sample-response to a micronutrient intervention. *Nutrients* 10(2): 152. https://doi.org/10.3390/nu10020152.

[59] Opie, R.S., O'Neil, A., Jacka, F.N. et al. (2017) A modified Mediterranean dietary intervention for adults with major depression: Dietary protocol and feasibility data from the SMILES trial. *Nutritional Neuroscience* 21(7): 487–501. https://doi.org/10.1080/1028415X.2017.1312841.

[60] Cope, E.C., and Levenson, C.W. (2010) Role of zinc in the development and treatment of mood disorders. *Current Opinion in Clinical Nutrition and Metabolic Care* 13(6): 685–689. https://doi.org/10.1097/MCO.0b013e32833df61a.

[61] Weinberg Levin, S., & Gattari, T.B. (2023) Iron deficiency in psychiatric patients. *Current Psychiatry* 22(3): 25–29. https://doi.org/10.12788/cp.0337.

[62] Field, D.T., Cracknell, R.O., Eastwood, J.R. et al. (2022) High-dose vitamin B_6 supplementation reduces anxiety and strengthens visual surround suppression. *Human Psychopharmacology: Clinical and Experimental* 37(6): e2852. https://doi.org/10.1002/hup.2852.

63 https://www.mdpi.com/2072-6643/15/17/3859

64 https://stacks.cdc.gov/view/cdc/3526

65 Anglin, R.E., Samaan, Z., Walter, S.D., & McDonald, S.D. (2013) Vitamin D deficiency and depression in adults: Systematic review and meta-analysis. *British Journal of Psychiatry* 202: 100–107. https://doi.org/10.1192/bjp.bp.111.106666.

66 https://www.ncbi.nlm.nih.gov/pmc/articles/PMC9864223/#B77-pharmaceuticals-16-00130

67 Cussotto, S., Delgado, I., Oriolo, G. et al. (2022) Low omega-3 polyunsaturated fatty acids predict reduced response to standard antidepressants in patients with major depressive disorder. *Depression and Anxiety* 39(5): 407–418. https://doi.org/10.1002/da.23257.

68 https://www.health.harvard.edu/mind-and-mood/omega-3s-for-anxiety

69 https://www.sciencedirect.com/science/article/pii/S0952327823000418#sec0014

70 Zhang, W.Y., Guo, Y.J., Han, W.X. et al. (2019) Curcumin relieves depressive-like behaviors via inhibition of the NLRP3 inflammasome and kynurenine pathway in rats suffering from chronic unpredictable mild stress. *International Immunopharmacology* 67: 138–144. https://doi.org/10.1016/j.intimp.2018.12.012.

71 Roohi-Azizi, M., Arabzadeh, S., Amidfar, M. et al. (2017) Citicoline combination therapy for major depressive disorder: A randomized, double-blind, placebo-controlled trial. *Clinical Neuropharmacology* 40(1): 1–5. https://doi.org/10.1097/WNF.0000000000000185.

72 Singh, P., Gollapalli, K., Mangiola, S. et al. (2023) Taurine deficiency as a driver of aging. *Science* 380(6649). https://doi.org/10.1126/science.abn9257.

73 Palatnik, A., Frolov, K., Fux, M., & Benjamin J. (2001) Double-blind, controlled, crossover trial of inositol versus fluvoxamine for the treatment of panic disorder. *Journal of Clinical Psychopharmacology* 21(3): 335–339. https://doi.org/10.1097/00004714-200106000-00014.

74 https://restorativemedicine.org/library/monographs/berberine/

75 https://www.ncbi.nlm.nih.gov/pmc/articles/PMC10604532/

76 Nagano, M., Shimizu, K., Kondo, R. et al. (2010) Reduction of depression and anxiety by 4 weeks *Hericium erinaceus* intake. Biomedical Research 31(4):

231–237. https://doi.org/10.2220/biomedres.31.231.

[77] http://www.stevenraker.com/Cordyceps_Ascomycetes.pdf

[78] Siddiqui, S.A., Ali Redha, A., Snoeck, E.R. et al. (2022) Anti-depressant properties of crocin molecules in saffron. *Molecules* 27(7): 2076. https://doi.org/10.3390/molecules27072076.

[79] Johnson, K.V.-A., & Laura Steenbergen, L. (2022) Gut feelings: Vagal stimulation reduces emotional biases. *Neuroscience* 494: 119–131. https://doi.org/10.1016/j.neuroscience.2022.04.026.

[80] Trivedi, G., Sharma, K., Saboo, B. et al. (2023) Humming (simple bhramari pranayama) as a stress buster: A Holter-based study to analyze heart rate variability (HRV) parameters during bhramari, physical activity, emotional stress, and sleep. *Cureus* 15(4): e37527. https://doi.org/10.7759/cureus.37527.

[81] https://www.sciencedaily.com/releases/2019/04/190412094728.htm

[82] https://www.ted.com/talks/matt_walker_sleep_is_your_superpower?language=en

[83] https://www.nih.gov/news-events/nih-research-matters/lack-sleep-disrupts-brains-emotional-controls

[84] De Weerdt, S. (2022) Can resetting the body clock help with depression? *Nature*, 24 August. https://www.nature.com/articles/d41586-022-02211-y.

[85] https://www.youtube.com/watch?v=h9HpDQN6Cqc

[86] Pearce, M., Garcia, L., Abbas, A. et al. (2022) Association between physical activity and risk of depression: A systematic review and meta-analysis. *JAMA Psychiatry* 79(6): 550–559. https://doi.org/10.1001/jamapsychiatry.2022.0609.

[87] Matthieu, C., Philippe, G., Alexis, M., & Marion, L. (2021) Interplay between exercise and gut microbiome in the context of human health and performance. *Frontiers in Nutrition* 8: 637010. https://doi.org/10.3389/fnut.2021.637010.

[88] Gordon, B.R., McDowell, C.P., Hallgren, M. et al. (2018) Association of efficacy of resistance exercise training with depressive symptoms: Meta-analysis and meta-regression analysis of randomized clinical trials. *JAMA Psychiatry* 75(6): 566–576. https://doi.org/10.1001/jamapsychiatry.2018.0572.

[89] Agudelo, L.Z., Femenía, T., Orhan, F. et al. (2014) Skeletal muscle PGC-1a1 modulates kynurenine metabolism and mediates resilience to stress-induced depression. *Cell* 159(1): 33–45. https://doi.org/10.1016/j.cell.2014.07.051.

[90] https://nature.com/articles/s4157

[91] Singh, B., Olds, T., Curtis, R. et al. (2023) Effectiveness of physical activity interventions for improving depression, anxiety and distress: An overview of systematic reviews. *British Journal of Sports Medicine* 57: 1203–1209. https://doi.org/10.1136/bjsports-2022-106195.

STEPHANIE J MOORE